DIY
Braids

DIY
Braids

From Crowns to Fishtails,
Easy, Step-by-Step
Hair-Braiding Instructions

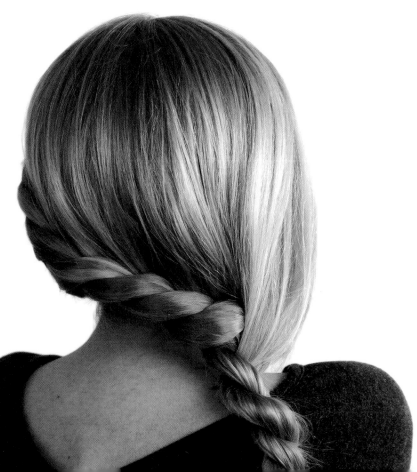

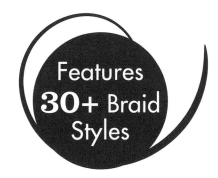

Features
30+ Braid
Styles

SASHA COEFIELD

Creator of the Beauty YouTube
Channel asksash88

Published by
Adams Media, a division of F+W Media, Inc.
57 Littlefield Street, Avon, MA 02322. U.S.A.
www.adamsmedia.com

ISBN 10: 1-4405-6739-5
ISBN 13: 978-1-4405-6739-1
eISBN 10: 1-4405-6740-9
eISBN 13: 978-1-4405-6740-7

Printed in the United States of America.

10 9 8 7 6 5 4 3 2 1

Readers are urged to take all appropriate precautions before undertaking any how-to task. Always read and follow instructions and safety warnings for all tools and materials, and call in a professional if the task stretches your abilities too far. Although every effort has been made to provide the best possible information in this book, neither the publisher nor the author is responsible for accidents, injuries, or damage incurred as a result of tasks undertaken by readers. This book is not a substitute for professional services.

Many of the designations used by manufacturers and sellers to distinguish their product are claimed as trademarks. Where those designations appear in this book and F+W Media was aware of a trademark claim, the designations have been printed with initial capital letters.

Cover and interior photographs by Sasha Coefield.

This book is available at quantity discounts for bulk purchases.
For information, please call 1-800-289-0963.

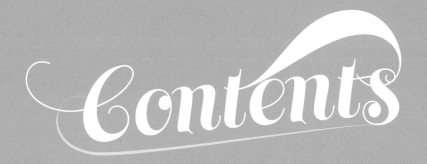

Contents

INTRODUCTION

Creating amazing braid designs is not only fun, it's incredibly easy with just a few simple tools. It really requires no experience, and instantly adds a personal touch to any hairstyle. You just need to learn about a few basic tools and master the most basic braids to get the best results and achieve the hair designs in this book.

The most important thing to remember is this: Practice makes perfect. You shouldn't get discouraged if your first braid doesn't come out exactly like the picture. While many of the hairstyles in this book are simple, others require a lot more braiding experience or a solid understanding of different braiding styles. But don't worry—after a few tries and with the right tools, you'll master these intricate braids and even be able to create your own original ones.

So say goodbye to boring hairstyles that leave you wanting more, and hello to attention-grabbing braids! With this book, you'll have everything you need to turn uninspired hair into fun, one-of-a-kind styles.

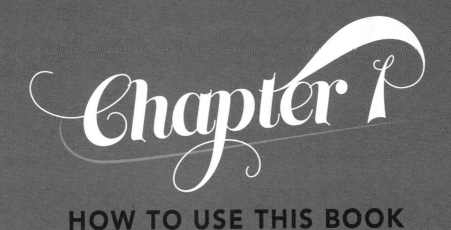

Chapter 1

HOW TO USE THIS BOOK

You might think that hairstylists are the only ones who can create beautiful, intricate braids. After all, they've taken classes and have made a career out of giving thousands of clients the perfect style. But creating complex braids isn't nearly as difficult as you might think. In fact, once you get started, you'll wonder why you were ever intimidated by the designs you see in magazines and online. Best of all, you'll have the satisfaction of knowing that not only did you accomplish this salon-quality look on your own, but you didn't have to spend a lot of money doing so. There are just a couple of things you need to know before you get started.

Prepping Your Hair for Creating Braids

In order to get the most beautiful braids possible, you will want to make sure you prep your hair according to what best suits your hair type. Most women will be able to create the styles in this book using dry hair, but if you are new to braiding, you may want to start off with damp hair. Dampening your hair with a spritz of water will make your hair more manageable, make the braids look sleeker, and help prevent the hairstyle from falling out. If you have very fine, straight hair that tends to loosen up in braids, applying mousse right before braiding may help braids stay in place and reduce flyaways. Those with curly hair will want to apply a smoothing serum or curl cream before braiding to avoid frizz. It may also be helpful for you to try out these braided hairstyles with unwashed hair since the oils in your hair will help you create tight, intricate-looking braids without having to use a lot of product.

Hair Tools

While every braid is different, there are a few things you should keep on hand when you're creating these intricate styles. Since many of the braids in this book require that you part your hair before you do anything else, you'll always want a comb close by to make sure that your part is even and that you can easily separate sections of hair. A comb will also come in handy for styles that require teasing the hair to create more volume. When securing a braid or ponytail, you'll want to use clear hair elastics or ones that match your hair color so they will be barely visible and will not distract from the hairstyle. Bobby pins are another item used throughout the book, and they will become your new best friends. Beauty supply stores often have higher quality bobby pins that will grip your hair better and hold the hairstyle in longer than the bobby pins you'll find at your local drug store. Many times people buy brown bobby pins by default, but you can find them in a range of colors to best match your hair tone. You may also want to finish all of the hairstyles in this book with a little hairspray, particularly if you have fine, sleek hair that falls out of hairstyles easily. The hairspray will help define your braids and ensure that the hairstyle lasts all day. No matter what tool you use, be sure to clean it after you finish the braid designs, especially if you're using hairspray, in order to extend its life and get a clean look every time.

Braiding Techniques

People always seem to feel the grass is greener on the other side when it comes to hair. But the truth is, braids lend themselves to a variety of hair colors and textures, so don't dismiss a hairstyle simply because you don't think it could work on your hair type. Curly hair, for instance, works beautifully with these styles because it adds to the messy, bohemian vibe that braids naturally lend themselves to. If you find that one hairstyle doesn't suit you quite well, feel free to change it around, such as by parting your hair differently or adding a bit of texture to it. Get creative and have fun! Let these hairstyles provide you with inspiration to create your own and adjust them to best fit your face shape, style, and preferences.

If you try out a hairstyle and really don't think it looks good with your hair because it's too thick or too thin, consider increasing or reducing the amount of hair incorporated into the braid. If you are not happy with your hair texture for a particular style, use a flat iron to make your hair sleek and straight, or add volume and dimension with a curling iron. A quick fix for hair that doesn't have the length or thickness you desire is to add a few clip-in hair extensions. These can really help make braids look luscious and beautiful without any long-term commitment.

Basic Braids

The Regular and Reverse Three-Stranded Braids are the basis for learning many of the other braids in this book. While they may look similar, they use slightly different techniques. With the Regular Three-Stranded Braid, you take the strands from the outside and place them *over* the middle section as you braid. This technique is utilized in the French braid. When braiding the Reverse Three-Stranded Braid, you take the outside strands and place them *under* the middle strand as you braid. This technique of braiding under is used in the Dutch braid.

Regular Three-Stranded Braid

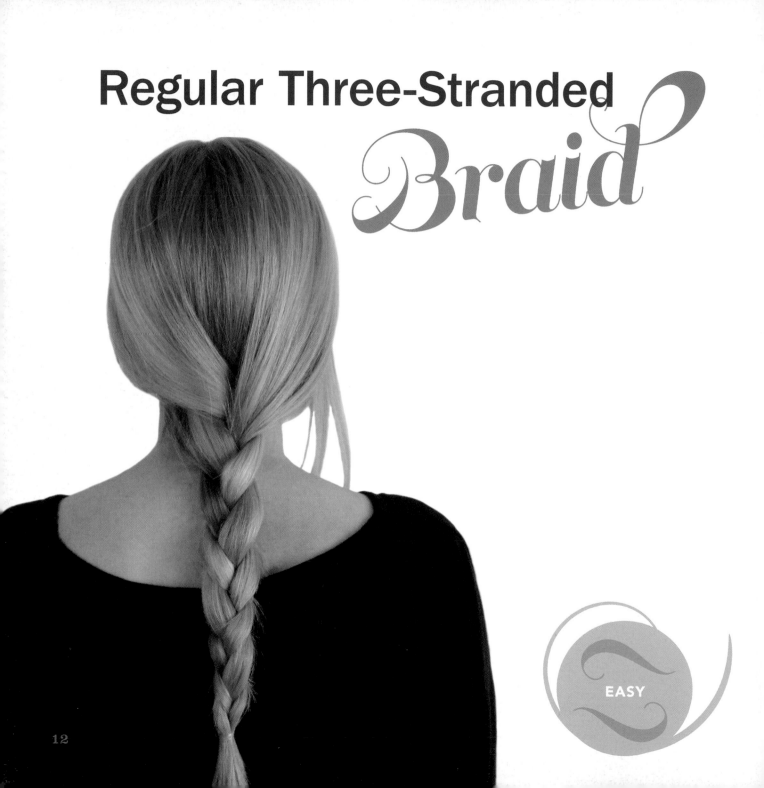

EASY

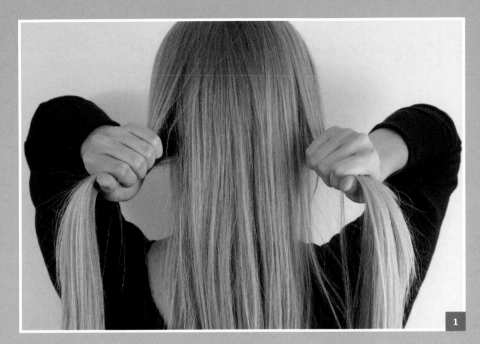

1. Begin by dividing your hair into three sections.

2. Place the left strand *over* the middle strand. The section that was on the left is now in the middle.

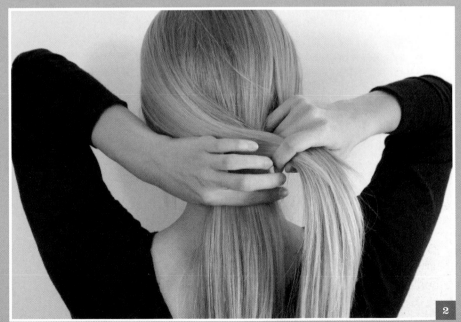

3. Next, place the right section *over* the middle section.

4. Now go back to the left side and place the left strand over the middle strand.

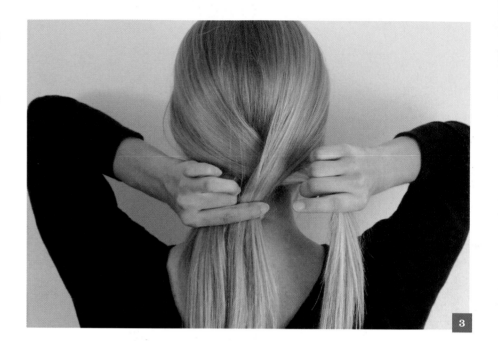

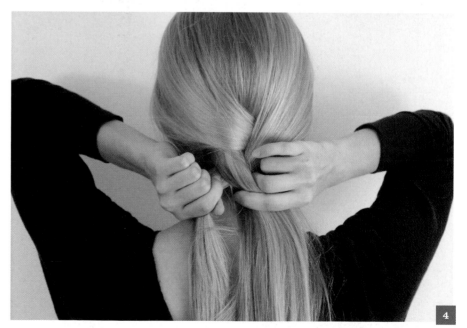

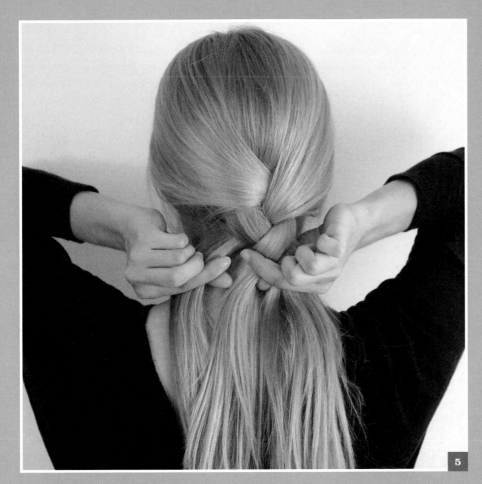

5. Place the right section over the middle section. Continue alternating between the left side and right side until you have reached the ends of your hair. Make sure to place the outer strands over the middle strand. Secure the braid with a hair tie.

Reverse Three-Stranded *Braid*

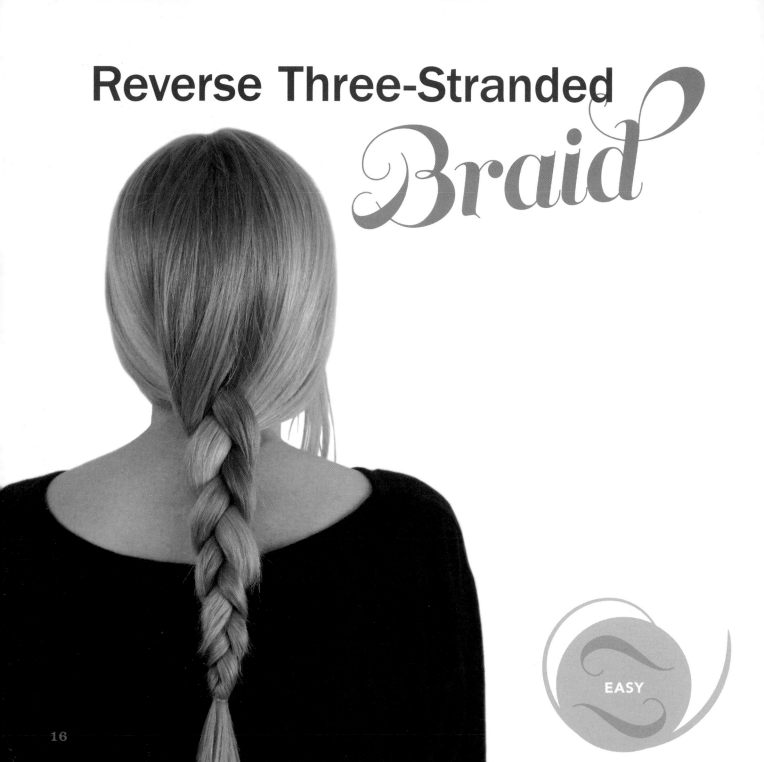

EASY

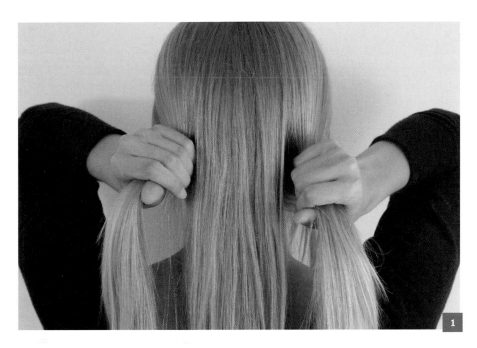

1. Divide your hair into three sections.

2. Place the left strand *under* the middle strand. The strand that was on the left is now in the middle.

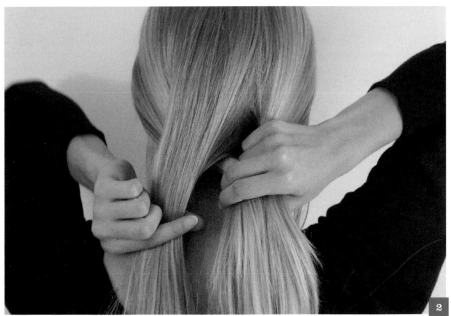

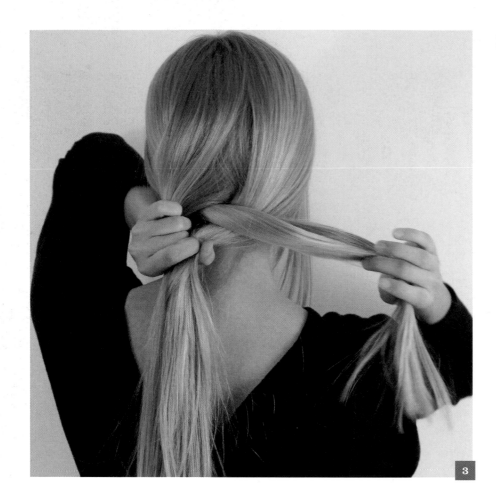

3. Take the strand on the right and place it *under* the strand in the middle. Continue alternating between the left and right sides until you have reached the ends of your hair. Make sure to place the outer strands under the middle strand. Secure the braid with a hair tie.

Chapter 2

BRAIDED STYLES

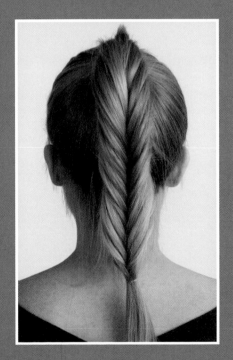
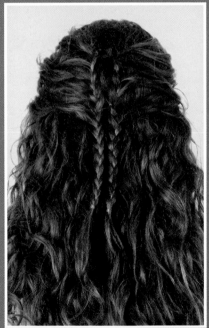
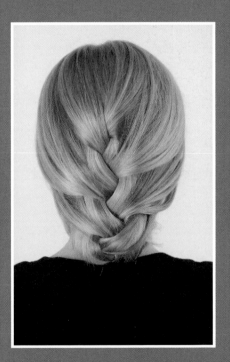

Tucked French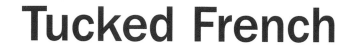

Forget the '80s with its poofy bangs, scrunchies, and boring French braids—this look puts a modern spin on the classic braid. In just a few easy steps, you can transform the outdated braid into a sophisticated hairstyle perfect for a date or just a night out on the town with the girls.

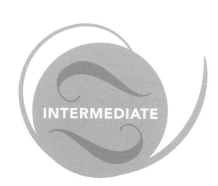
INTERMEDIATE

1. Gather a section of hair at the back of your head as if you were putting the top half of your hair up into a ponytail.

2. Divide the section into three smaller sections.

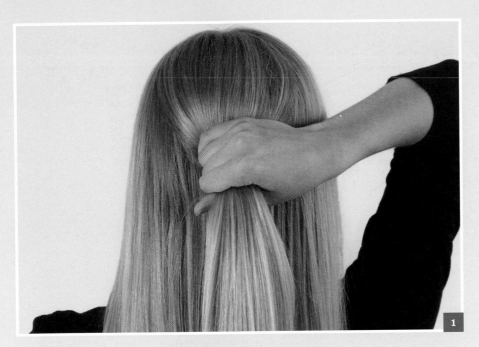

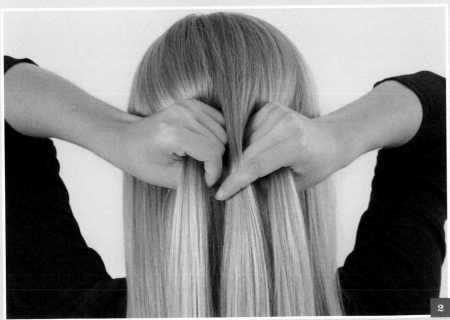

3. Take the right section and cross it over the middle section.

4. Take the left section and cross it over the middle section.

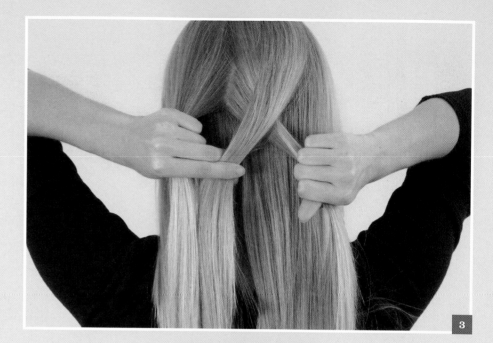

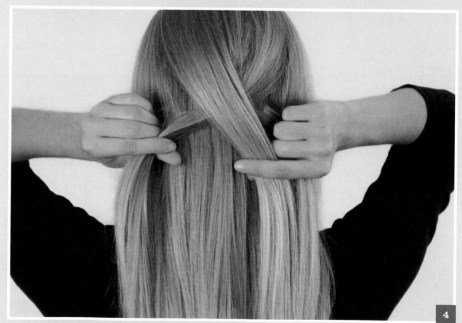

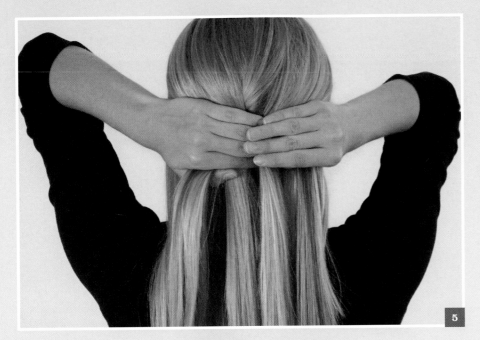

5. Begin French braiding the remaining hair by grabbing a new section of hair and adding it to the rightmost strand.

6. Take the new right section and cross it over the middle section.

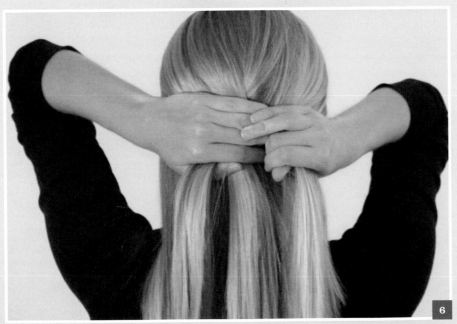

7. Gather hair from the left side of your head and add it to the leftmost strand.

8. Take the new left section and cross it over the middle section.

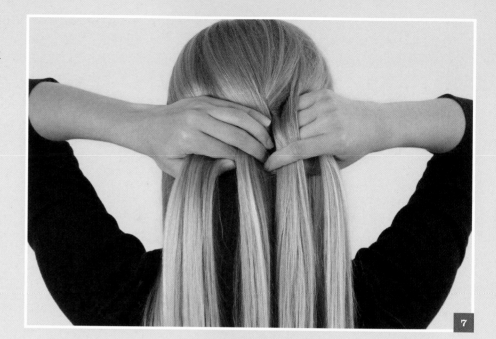

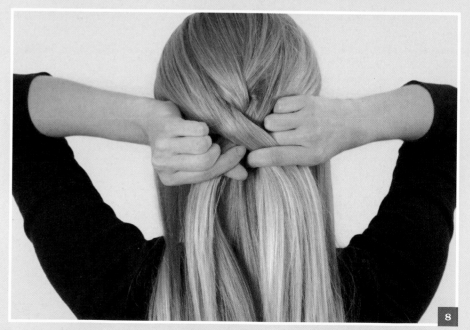

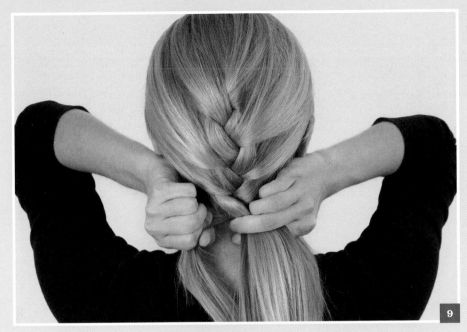

9. Continue French braiding until all of the hair closest to the scalp is incorporated into the braid. Then braid the remaining hair using the Regular Three-Stranded Braid technique.

10. Secure the braid with an elastic.

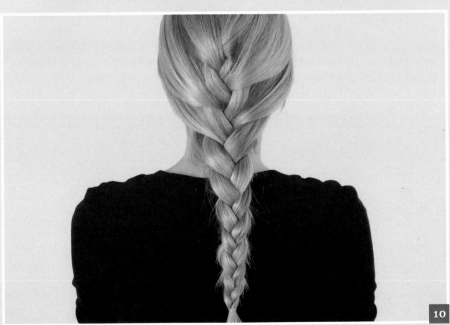

11. Roll the braid up towards the nape of your neck until all of it is tucked under the section of hair where your braid starts. Use bobby pins to secure the rolled-up braid against your head.

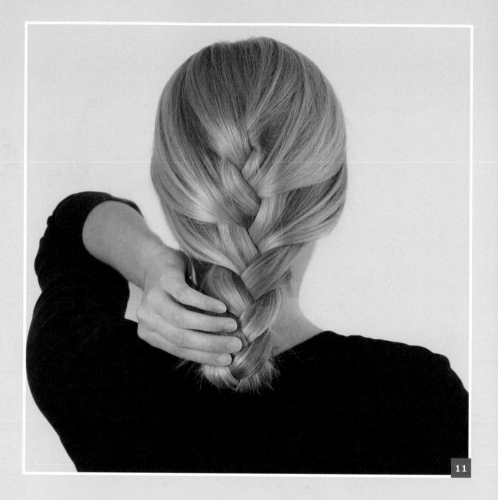

11

Fishtail *Braid*

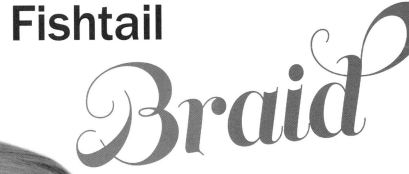

Once you get the hang of the Fishtail Braid, you can use the style to turn an everyday, boring hairstyle into a chic and interesting look. While they may appear very complex, Fishtail Braids are actually quite easy to accomplish. Keep in mind that the smaller the sections you use to create the braid, the more intricate and beautiful the hairstyle will be.

INTERMEDIATE

1. Secure your hair into a ponytail.

2. Divide the ponytail in half.

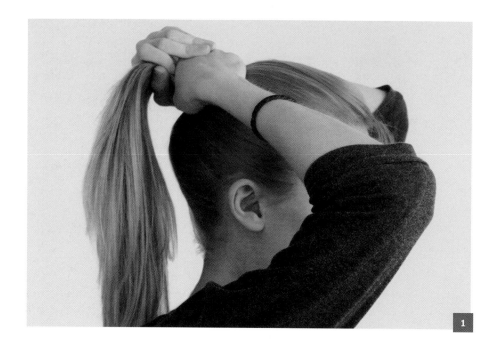

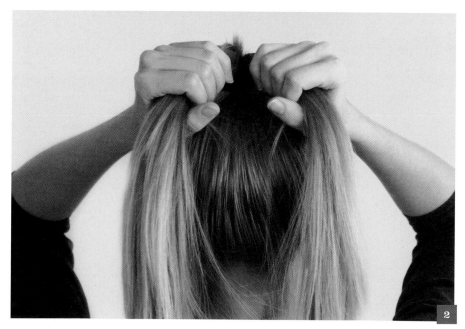

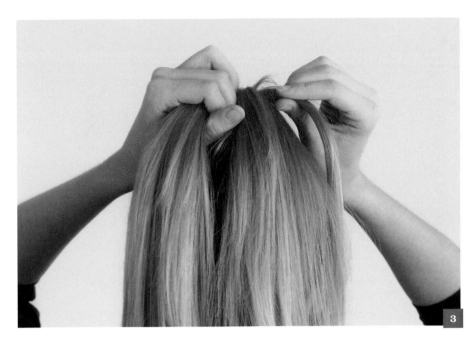

3. Take a very small piece of hair from the right section. The smaller the pieces of hair you use the more beautiful the braid will turn out.

4. Bring the small piece of hair over to the left section.

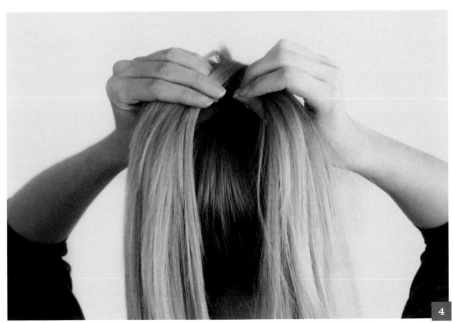

5. Now take a small section from the left and bring it over to the right section of hair.

6. Repeat Steps 2–3. Make sure to continually pull the braid tight so that it keeps its form as you are braiding.

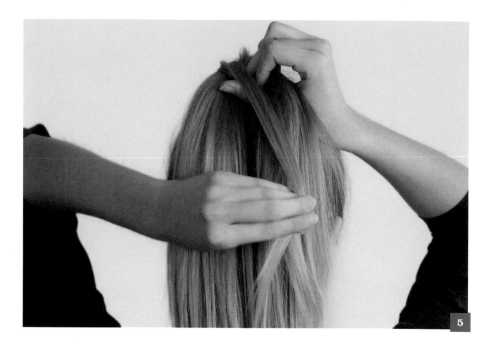

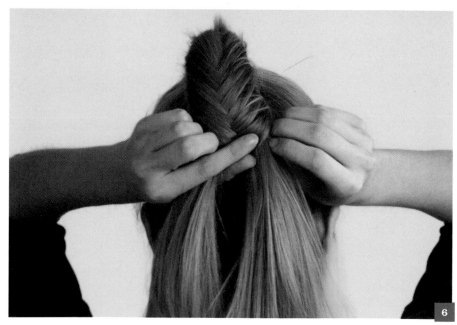

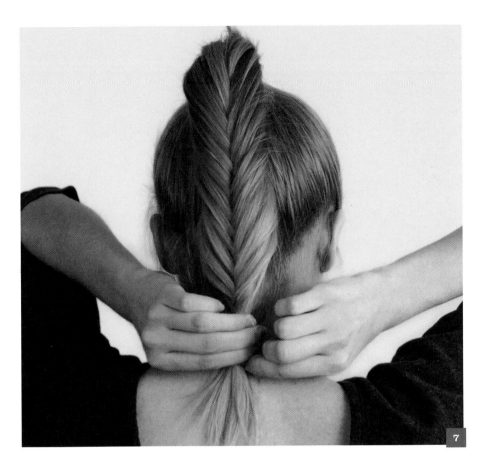

7. Continue braiding until you reach the ends of your hair, then secure your braid with a hair tie.

Lace
Braid

The best way to think about a Lace Braid is that it's a distant relative of the French braid. As with the popular hairstyle, you'll need to add additional sections of hair to one side as you braid, but in this intricate design, you'll weave in a Regular Three-Stranded Braid to the other side. Simple yet striking, this braid is a perfect every-day look.

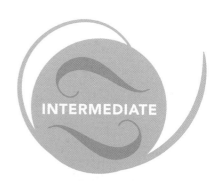

INTERMEDIATE

1. Take a small section of hair from one side of your head and divide it into three parts.

2. On the first round, gather the section on the right and put it over the section in the middle so that it is now the middle section.

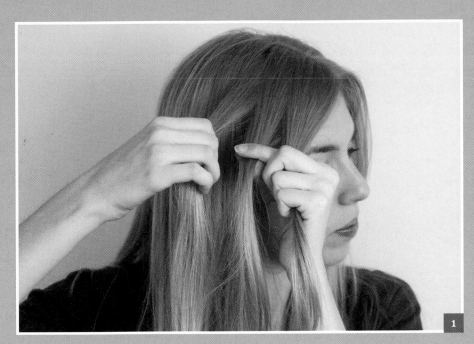

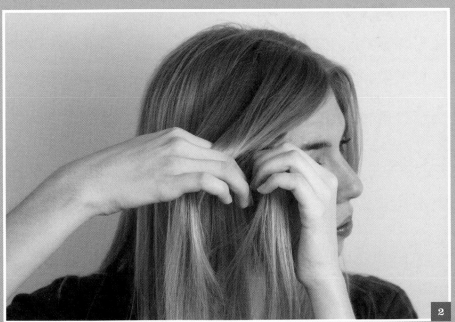

3. Take the section on the left and put it over the section in the middle.

4. On the second round, repeat Step 2 by taking the rightmost strand as is and placing it over the middle strand.

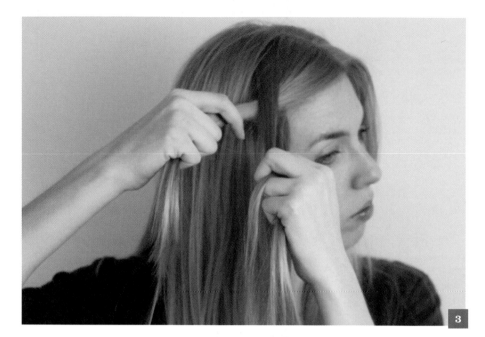

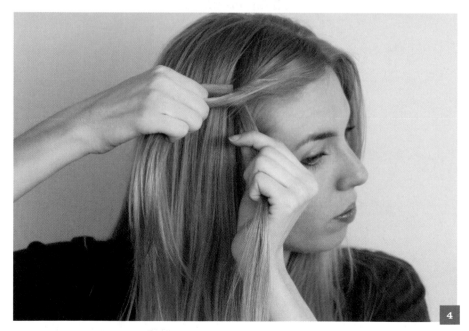

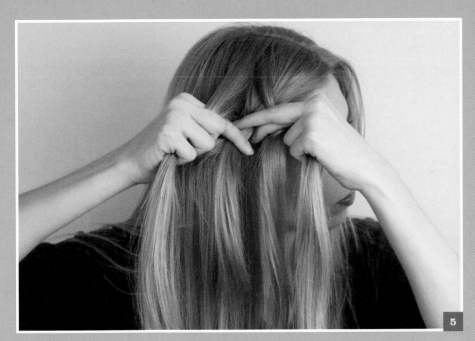

5. Take a small section from the rest of your hair and add it to the leftmost strand. Place this larger section over the middle strand.

6. Continue with this French braid modification, making sure to only add more sections of hair to the leftmost strand.

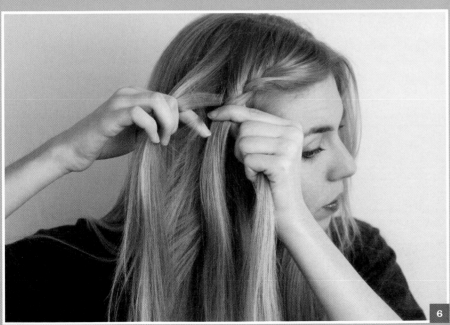

7. Continue braiding until you reach the ends of your hair, then secure your braid with a hair tie.

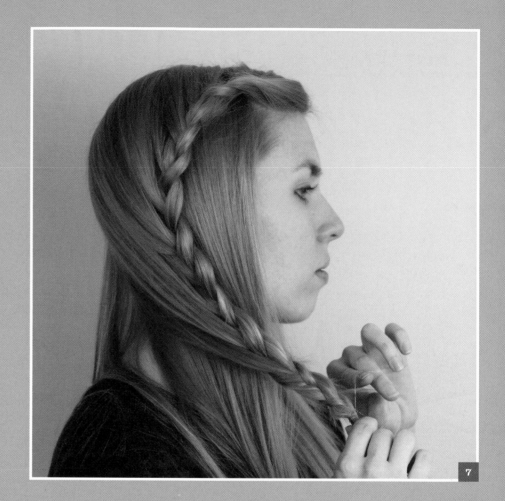

Dutch Braided *Headband*

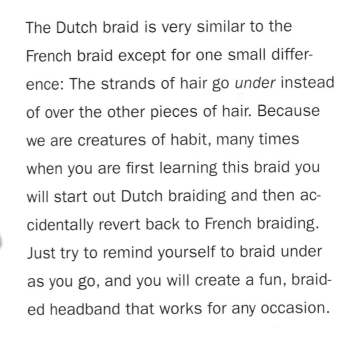

The Dutch braid is very similar to the French braid except for one small difference: The strands of hair go *under* instead of over the other pieces of hair. Because we are creatures of habit, many times when you are first learning this braid you will start out Dutch braiding and then accidentally revert back to French braiding. Just try to remind yourself to braid under as you go, and you will create a fun, braided headband that works for any occasion.

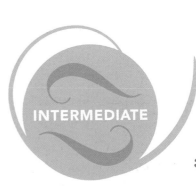

INTERMEDIATE

1. Gather a small section of hair from the front middle of your head.

2. Divide the hair into three sections with the first near your forehead and the other two behind it.

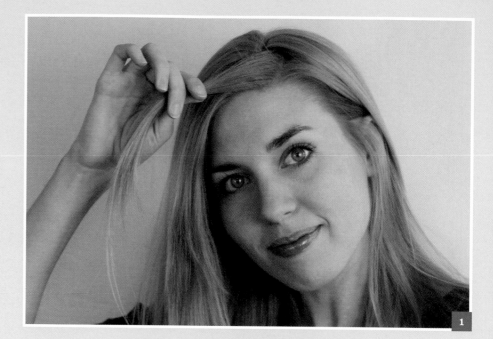

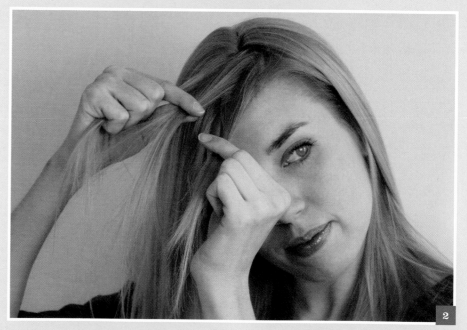

3. Take the section of hair on the right, closest to your forehead, and cross it *under* the middle section.

4. Take the left section and cross it underneath the section in the middle.

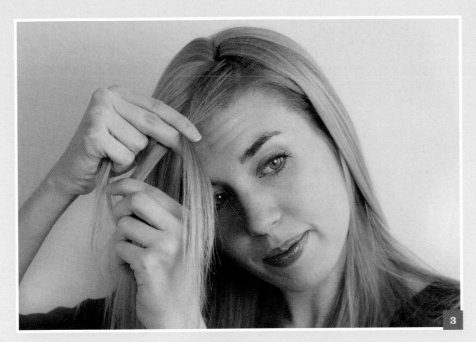

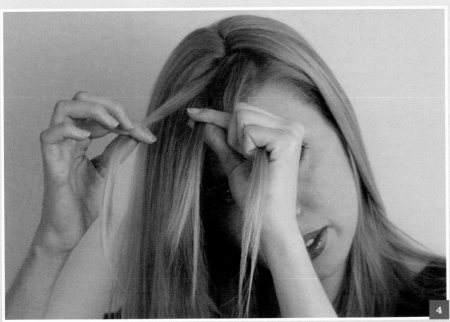

5. Now that you've started the Dutch braid, you will begin adding new hair as you braid. As you continue crossing the rightmost and leftmost sections underneath the middle one, make sure to add more strands of hair to these outer sections.

6. Continue Dutch braiding along your hairline.

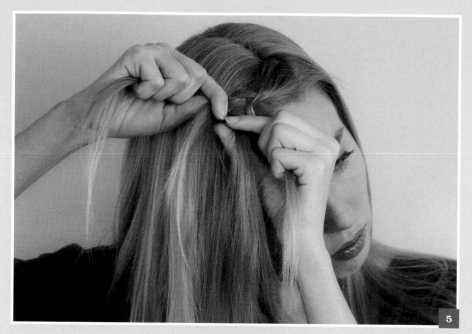

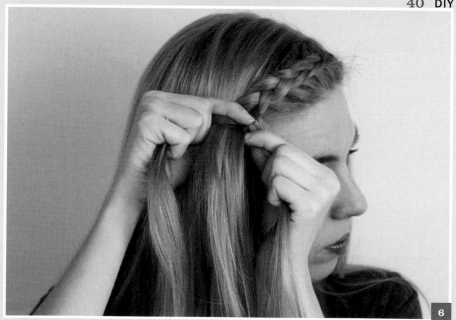

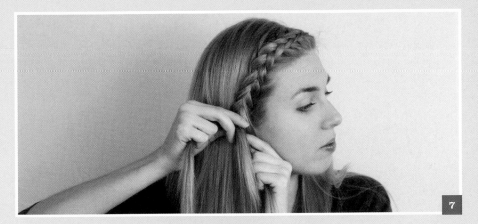

7. Once you have braided down to your ear, start creating a Reverse Three-Stranded Braid by simply crossing the right strand *under* the middle one and the left strand *under* the middle section. You no longer need to add more strands of hair to the outer sections.

8. Once you reach the ends of your hair, secure the braid with an elastic.

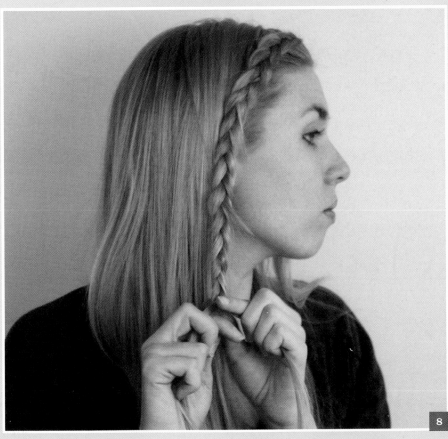

French Rope

Braid

Another eye-catching hairstyle, the French Rope Braid is an impressive do that is sure to have your friends asking how you created the look. While the style may look as if you've spent hours on it, it only takes a few minutes, so it's a great go-to for mornings when you're running late.

INTERMEDIATE

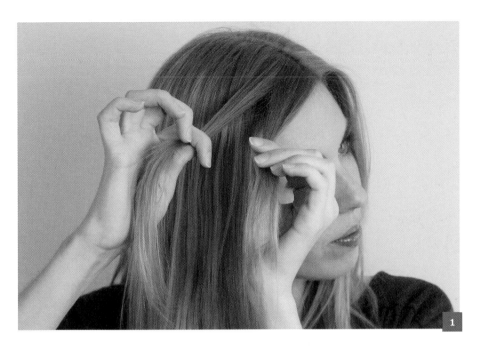

1. Gather a section of hair at the front of your head and divide it into two smaller sections.

2. Take the section in the front and cross it over the section behind it, bringing the back section to the front.

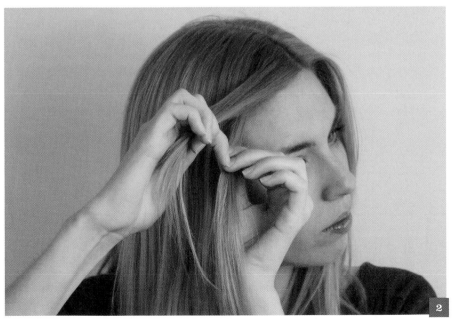

3. Add a small section of hair to the new front section.

4. Cross the front section over the back section and bring the back section forward.

5. Repeat Steps 2–4, adding new hair to the section in the front each time.

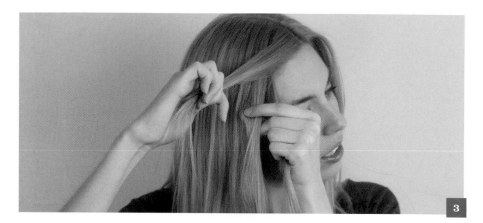

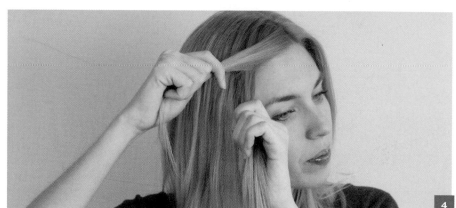

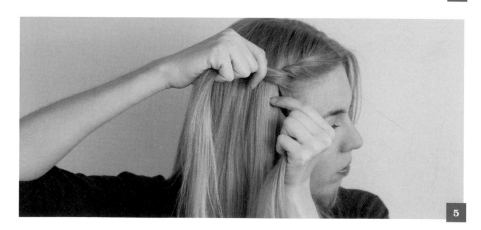

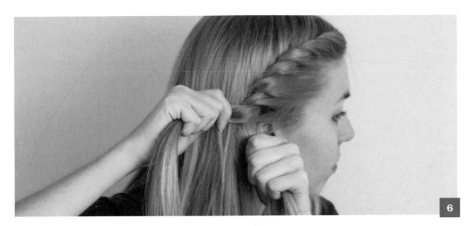

6. Continue until you have braided your hair to your liking.

7. Secure the braid with bobby pins.

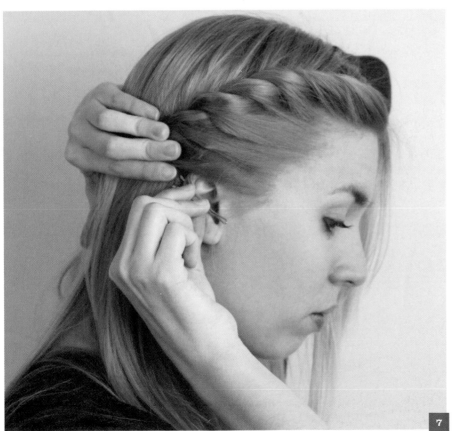

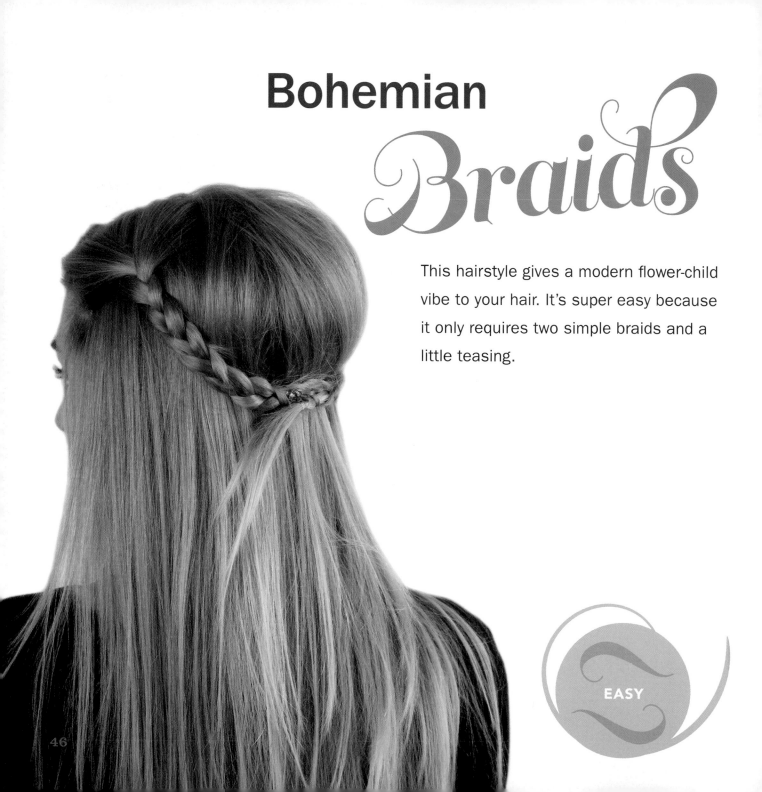

Bohemian

Braids

This hairstyle gives a modern flower-child vibe to your hair. It's super easy because it only requires two simple braids and a little teasing.

EASY

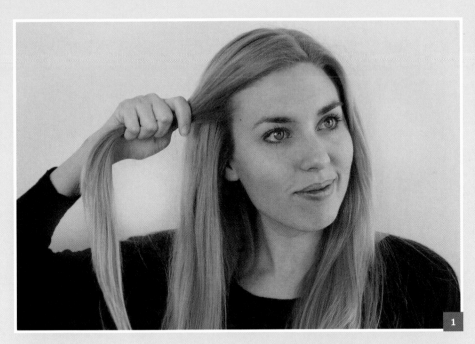

1. Take a medium-size section on one side of your head.

2. Do a Regular Three-Stranded Braid, making sure to braid heading towards the back of your head. This will ensure that the braid lies flat against your head when the style is completed. Secure the braid with a clear elastic.

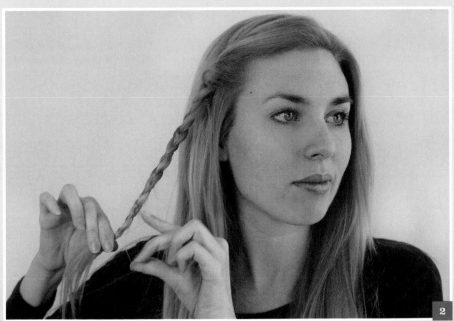

3. Repeat the same process on the other side.

4. At the crown of your head, grab and hold up a section of hair that is underneath the top layer of your hair and mist it with hairspray.

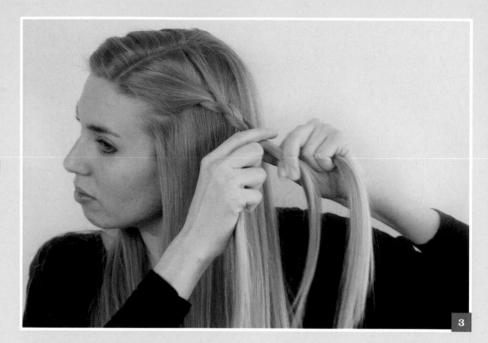

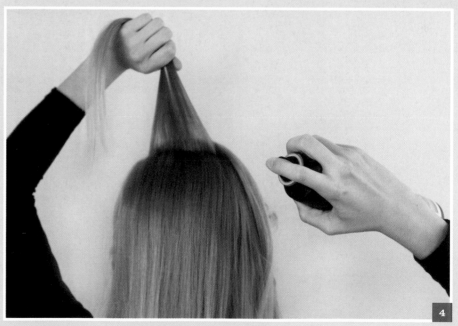

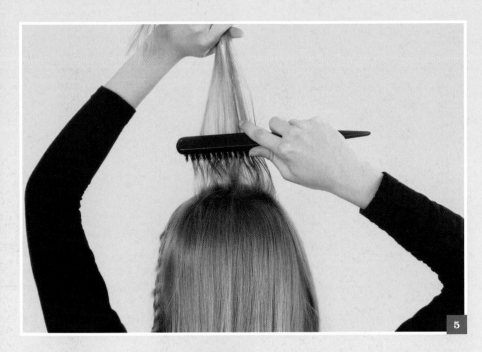

5. With a comb or teasing brush, brush the hair in a downward motion to tease this section of hair.

6. Repeat this process with a few more layers of hair below the section you just teased until you reach the desired amount of volume.

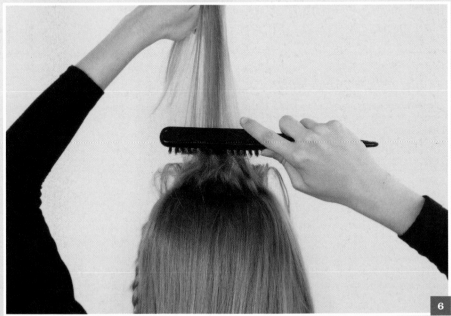

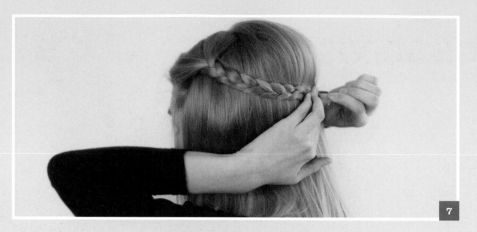

7. After you are done teasing, flip the hair back down and smooth out any teased parts that show through the top layer of hair. The hair at the crown of your head should be an even bump. Pin one braid below the teased hair with a few bobby pins.

8. Pin the second braid on top of the other braid, making an effort to hide the bobby pins inside the braids.

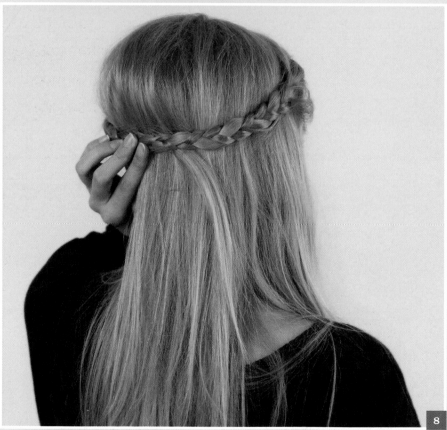

Crisscross *Braid*

Since it only takes a few minutes to master, the Crisscross Braid is one of the easiest braids to learn. However, the details in the finished product will leave others wondering how you created the delicate look.

EASY

1. Begin by separating a small section of hair at the nape of your neck from the rest of your hair.

2. Divide this section into two smaller sections of hair and divide one of those sections into two smaller strands. Wrap one strand around the left side of the rest of your hair and the other one around the right side.

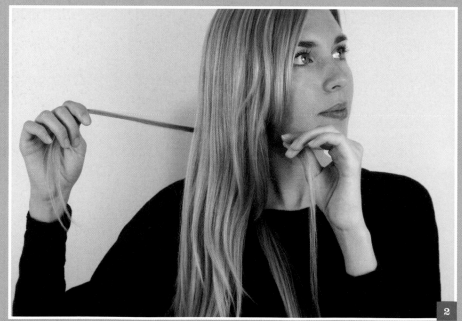

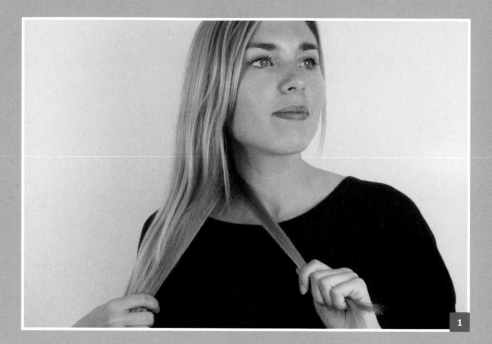

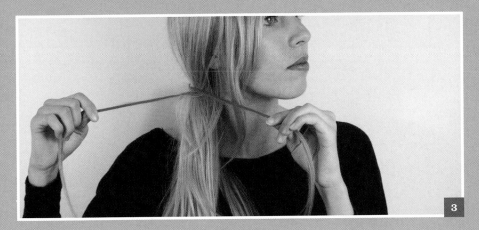

3. Cross the two strands over each other. The large section of untouched hair should look like a ponytail.

4. Cross the strands over each other under the ponytail.

5. Continue crossing the strands over and under the ponytail until you reach the ends of your ponytail. Secure with a hair tie.

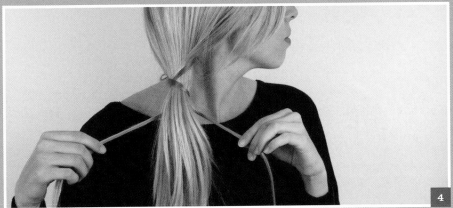

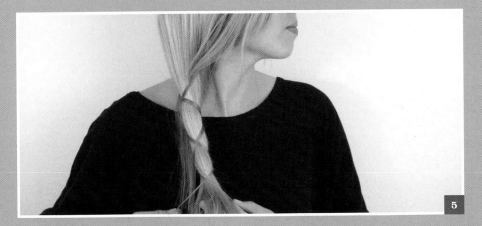

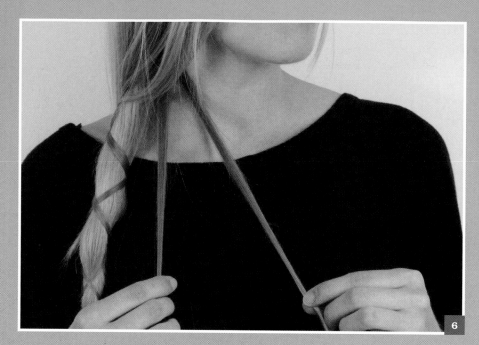

6. Repeat Steps 2–4 with your first section of hair. Make sure that when you cross the new strands, they cross above the first set of strands, so that the wrapped strands form a series of Xs. Secure with a hair tie.

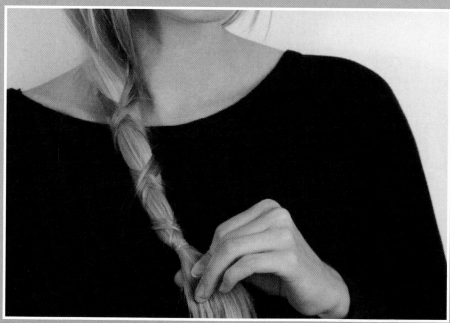

Double Braided

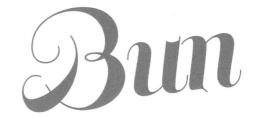

As the name suggests, the Double Braided Bun is simply just two Regular Three-Stranded Braids wrapped up into an elegant bun. If you wanted the hairstyle to be a bit more intricate, you could include more braids, but even just using two braids creates a gorgeous look.

EASY

1. Secure your hair into a ponytail and divide your ponytail into two sections. Take one section and divide it into three sections.

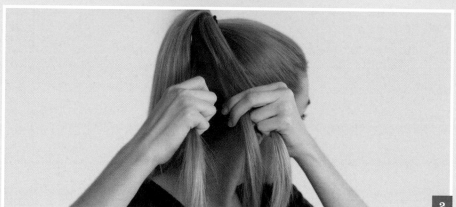

2. Take the section on the left and cross it with the section in the middle.

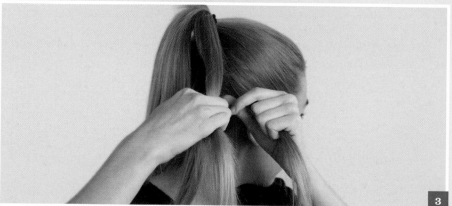

3. Now take the section on the right and cross it with the middle section.

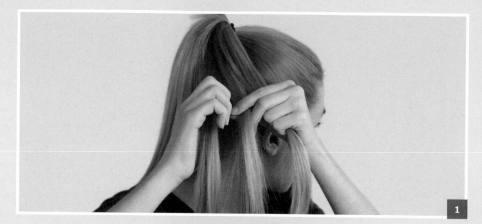

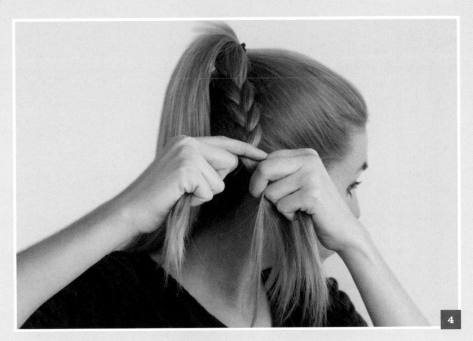

4. Continue braiding in this fashion until you reach the ends of your hair. This will give you a Regular Three-Stranded Braid.

5. Secure the braid with a hair tie.

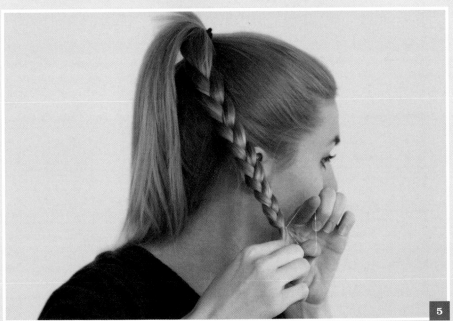

6. Take the remaining section of ponytail and create another Regular Three-Stranded Braid by repeating Steps 2–4.

7. Wrap one braid around the base of the other until you create a bun.

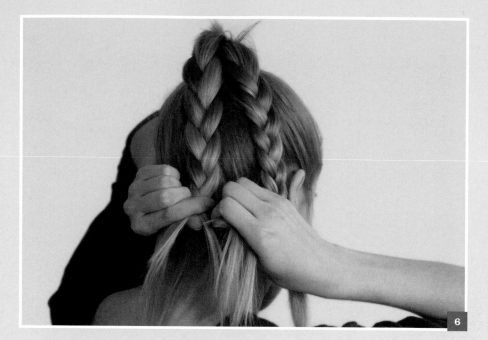

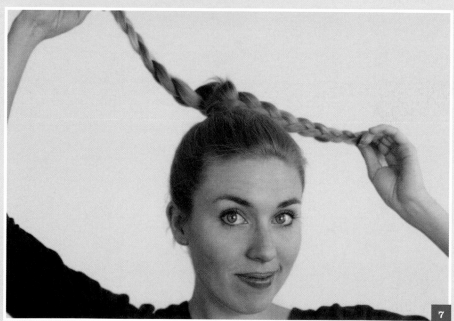

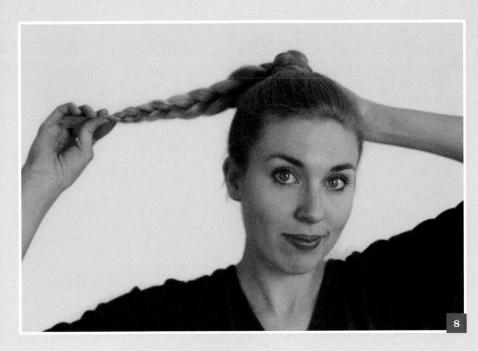

8. Secure your bun with a bobby pin.

9. Wrap the remaining braid around the bun and secure it with bobby pins.

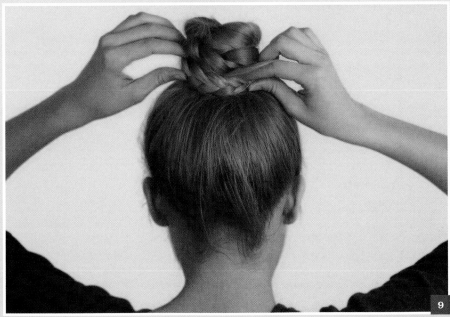

Braided *Bangs*

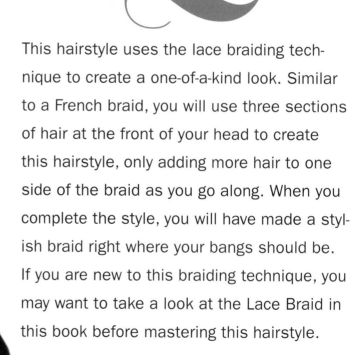

This hairstyle uses the lace braiding technique to create a one-of-a-kind look. Similar to a French braid, you will use three sections of hair at the front of your head to create this hairstyle, only adding more hair to one side of the braid as you go along. When you complete the style, you will have made a stylish braid right where your bangs should be. If you are new to this braiding technique, you may want to take a look at the Lace Braid in this book before mastering this hairstyle.

INTERMEDIATE

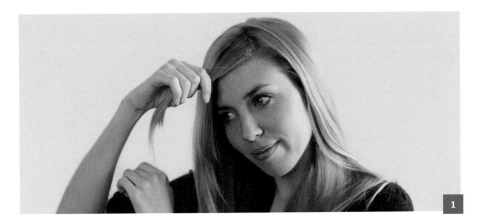

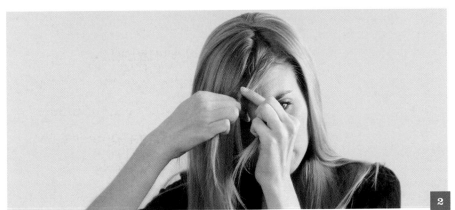

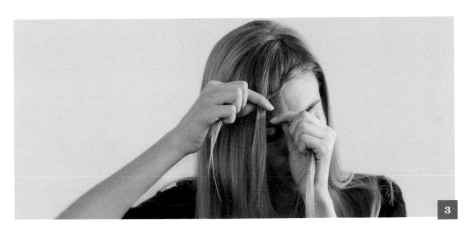

1. Part your hair to the side and gather a small section at the front of your head.

2. Begin French braiding your hair by separating it into three sections and then bringing the left section over the middle strands and then the right section over the middle strands.

3. Repeat the previous step, but add a small section of hair to the leftmost strand each time you move it over the middle strands. Do not add any hair to the rightmost strand while braiding.

4. Continue French braiding until you reach your ear.

5. Once you reach your ear, switch to a Regular Three-Stranded Braid and continue braiding until you reach the ends of your hair. Secure the braid with an elastic.

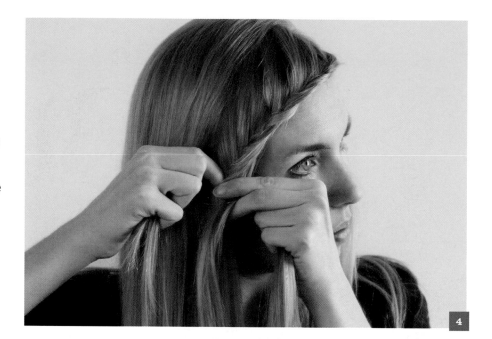

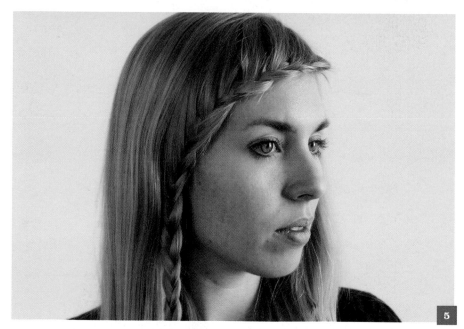

Waterfall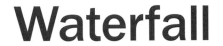

The Waterfall Braid is another unique braid that always leaves people wondering, "How did she do that?" The delicate way that your hair hangs after the design is completed makes it seem as if your hair is gently cascading down into place. By simply making a few tweaks to the French braid, you can achieve this whimsical hairstyle.

HARD

1. Gather a section of hair at the front of your head and divide it into three smaller sections.

2. Cross the section on the right over the section in the middle.

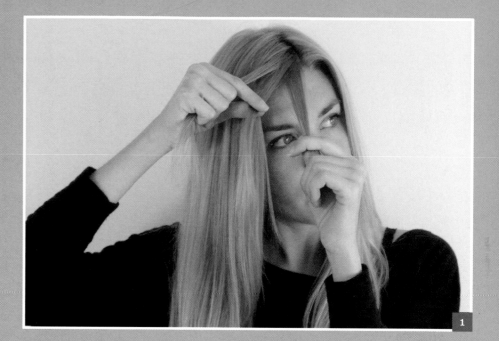

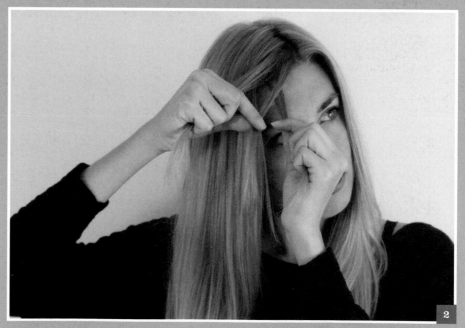

3. Cross the section on the left over the section in the middle.

4. Release the right section of hair.

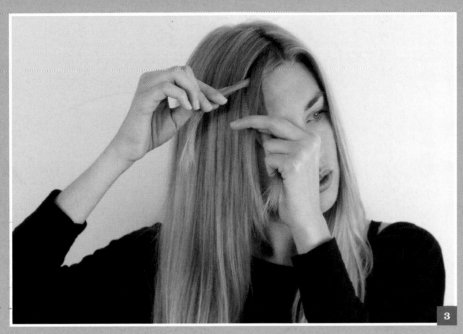

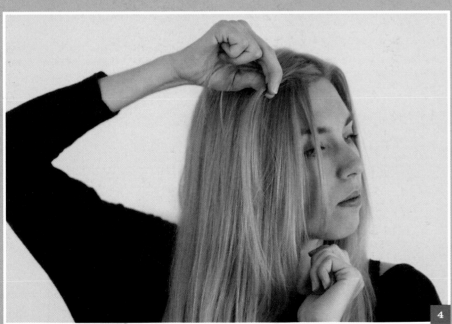

5. Pick up a new strand of hair behind the section of hair you released. This new strand will act as the new right section, which you will now cross over the middle section.

6. Add additional hair to the leftmost strand and place it over the middle section. You are treating the leftmost section like a normal French braid.

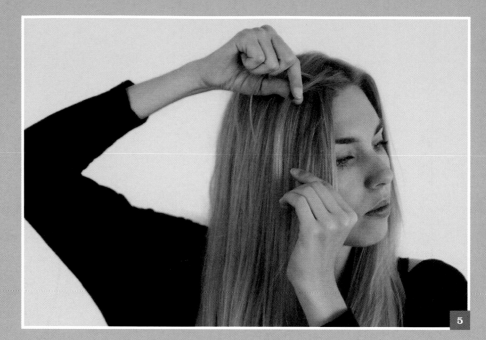

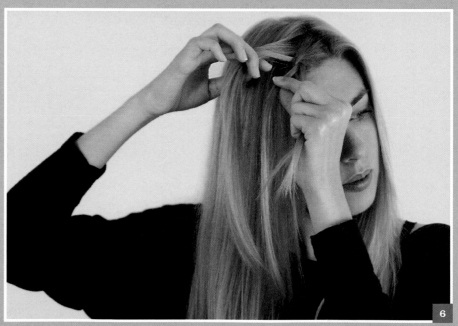

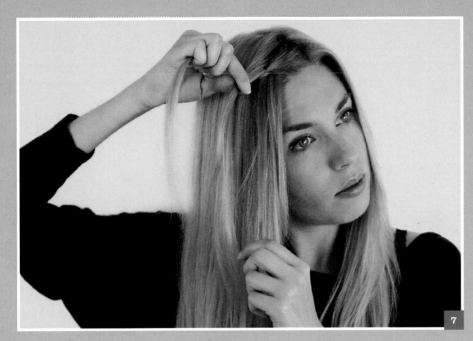

7. Release the right section of hair. Pick up a new strand behind it and put the new strand over the middle section.

8. Repeat Steps 6–7 until you have reached the back of your head. Secure the braid with bobby pins.

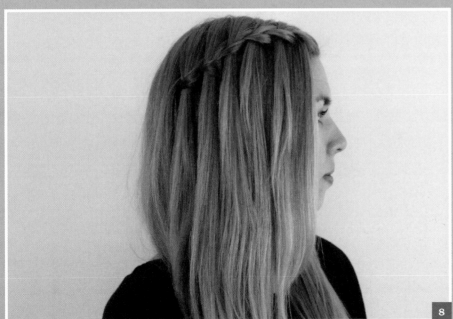

Snake
Braid

Chances are, you've never seen anything like the Snake Braid before. A far cry from the French braid, this interesting look seems complex, but is actually incredibly easy to create. To complete the hairstyle, all you will need to learn is the Regular Three-Stranded Braid technique and a few extra tricks to make it really stand out. Whether you tie it back or leave it hanging, you are guaranteed to turn heads no matter how you wear this braid!

EASY

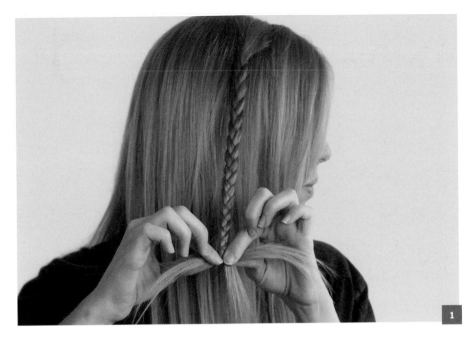

1. Take a medium-size section of hair from the center left side of your head and begin braiding it into a Regular Three-Stranded Braid by crossing the right section over the middle strands followed by the left section over the middle strands. It's best to avoid very small sections of hair for this hairstyle, particularly when you are first learning, because it makes the following steps more difficult to do. Also, make sure that you aren't braiding too tight or too loose.

2. Continue braiding until you reach the ends of your hair. Take the left and right sections and hold them together in one hand and hold the middle section with your other hand.

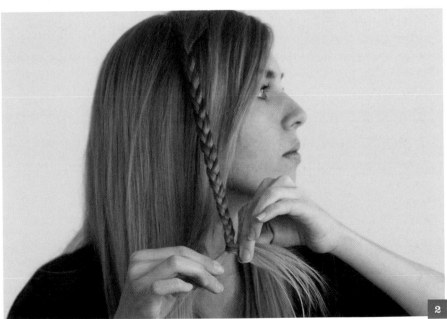

3. Use the hand that is holding the right and left sections to slide those pieces upwards towards the top of the braid while holding the middle section down with your other hand.

4. Continue sliding the braid upwards until it is compressed up at the top.

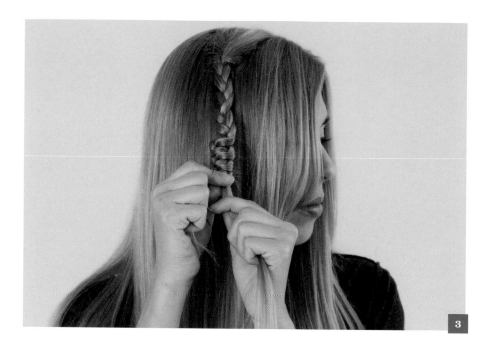

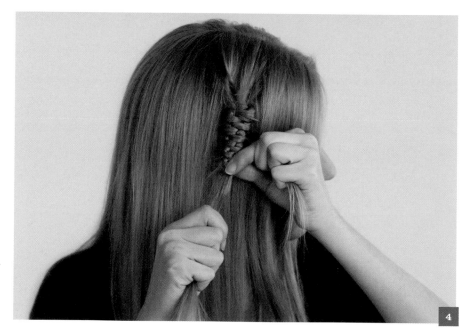

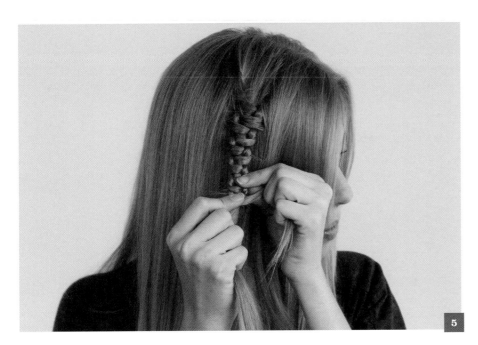

5. Pull the compressed braid back down a few inches.

6. Hold the bottom of the braid tightly in place with one hand while you even out the rest of the braid by sliding it up or down wherever it is uneven with the other hand.

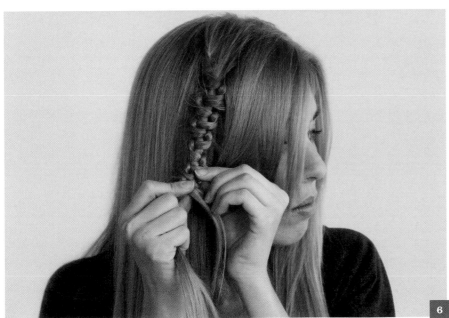

7. Secure the bottom of the braid, which should be about halfway down the length of your hair, with an elastic.

8. You can leave the braid as is or pin it back with a bobby pin for a slightly different look.

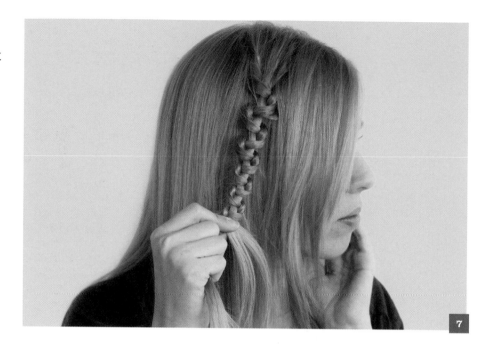

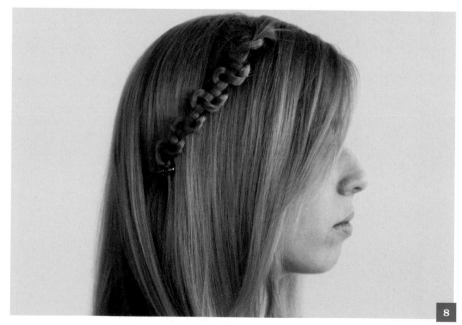

Triple Fishtail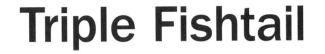

Just like it sounds, the Triple Fishtail Braid consists of three Fishtail Braids braided together into a single hair design. While this look may require some time and skill, the end result is worth the effort. Keep in mind that Fishtail Braids look their best when you use small sections of hair in your braids. Since this style can be difficult for beginners, you may want to master the regular Fishtail Braid found earlier in this book before trying your hand at this more complicated style.

HARD

73

1. Divide all of your hair into three sections.

2. Move the two outmost sections in front of your shoulders, so that you can focus on braiding the middle section. Divide this section in half.

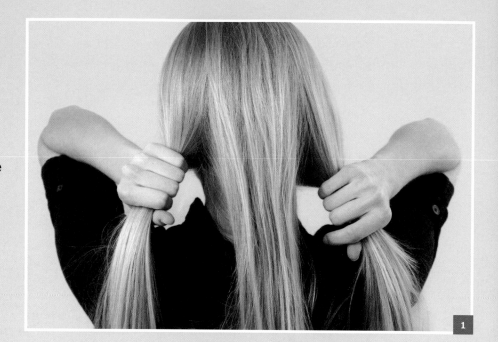

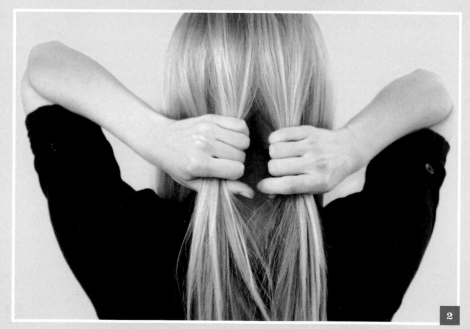

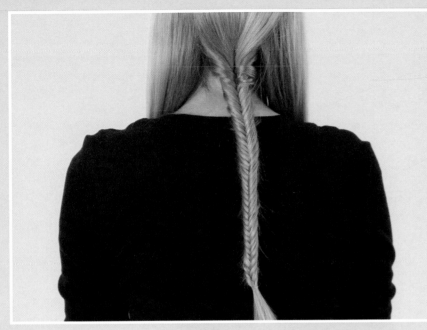

3. Begin fishtail braiding it by taking a very small piece of hair from the right section and bringing it over to the left section. Then take a small piece of hair from the section on the left and bring it over to the right section. Continue fishtail braiding until you reach the ends of your hair, then secure the braid with an elastic.

4. Once you have finished the middle Fishtail Braid, repeat the previous step with the left section of hair.

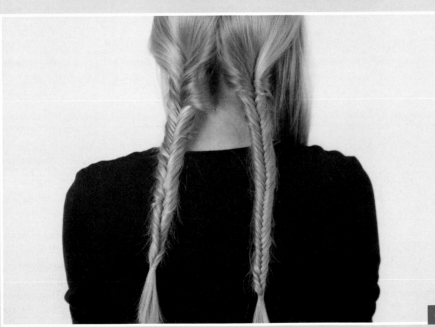

5. Once you have finished the second Fishtail Braid, repeat Step 3 with the remaining section of hair.

6. Take the braids you just created and treat them as you would if they were strands in a Regular Three-Stranded Braid. Cross the right Fishtail Braid over the middle one and then the left Fishtail Braid over the middle one.

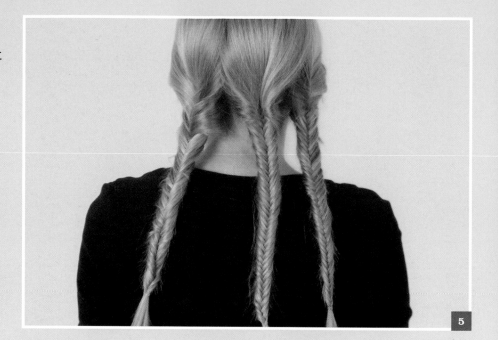

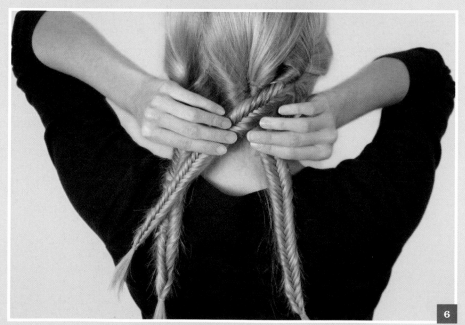

7. Continue this three-stranded braiding technique until you reach the ends of the braids.

8. Secure the braids together with an elastic.

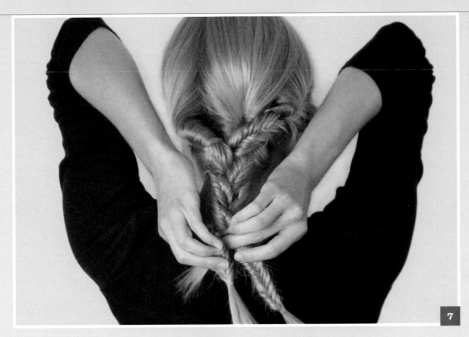

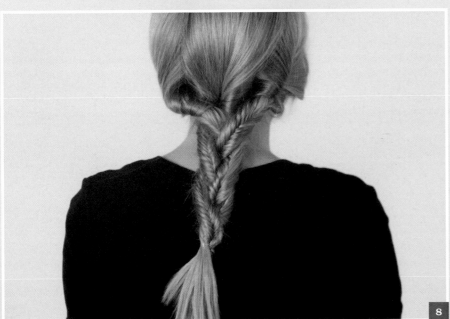

Knot
Braid

Elegant and refined, the Knot Braid is a simple braid that anyone can create. It utilizes the same technique that you use for the first step of tying your shoes where you cross your laces and tuck one underneath the other. However, the outcome is a beautiful updo that can be done in a matter of minutes and worn during special occasions.

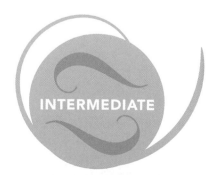

INTERMEDIATE

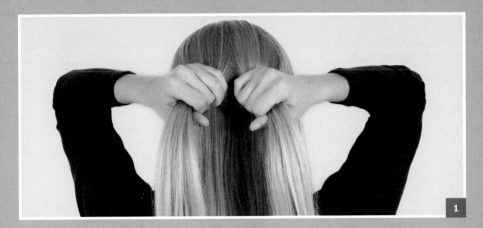

1. Separate your hair into two sections as if you were making a ponytail with the top half of your hair. Divide this top section into two smaller sections.

2. Cross the left section over and then underneath the right section. Weave the left section through the hole and pull on the ends of each section to tighten.

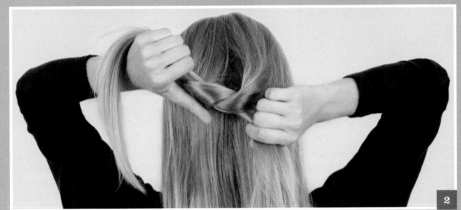

3. While still holding on to those sections, pick up new hair from the section of hair below the braid and add it to the hair in each of your hands. Repeat Step 2 with the new sections of hair. Using bigger or smaller sections of hair as you knot your hair will change the look of the braid.

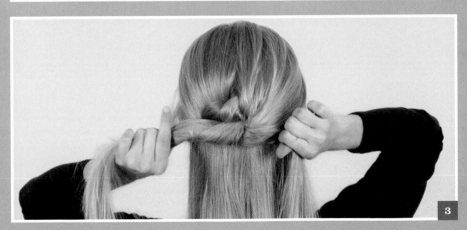

4. Continue creating knots until you have incorporated all your hair into the braid. Your braid should end around the nape of your neck.

5. Pull the ends tightly to ensure the hairstyle stays in place.

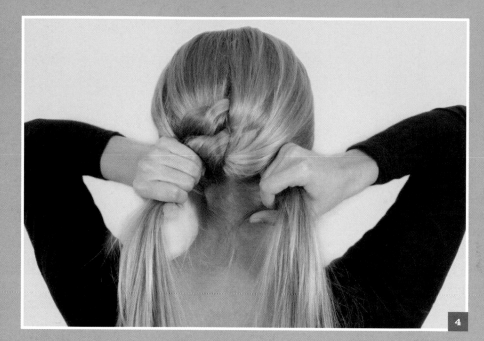

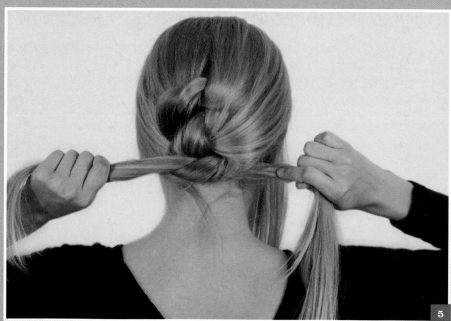

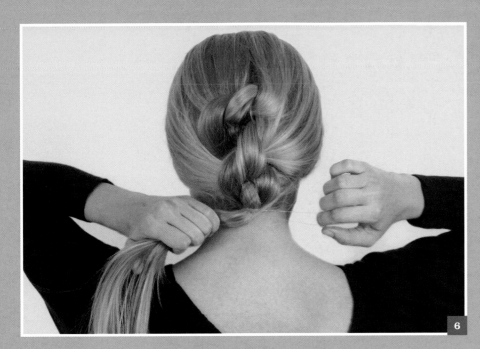

6. Secure the braid with an elastic.

7. Roll the excess hair into a bun and tuck it under the knot braid, using bobby pins to secure the hairstyle.

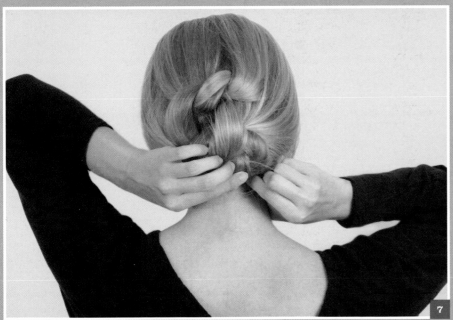

Dutch Braided
Spiral

A punched-up version of the Dutch braid, this look uses that technique to create a beautiful rose-like spiral at the back of your head. If you're still working on creating a Dutch braid, turn back to the Dutch Braided Headband for tips on perfecting this look. The intricate braid is stunning when pinned together and allows you to add decorative pins and headpieces to really make the look your own.

HARD

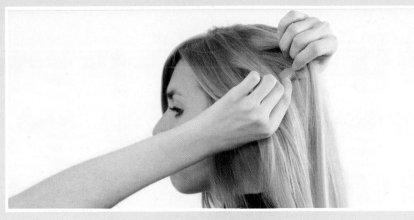

1. Divide the hair at the front of your head into three sections. Make sure to use medium-size sections when braiding since this hairstyle looks best with a bigger, chunkier braid.

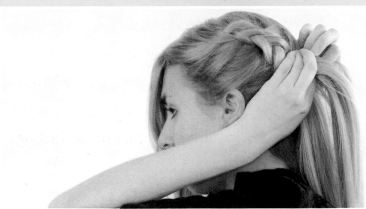

2. Start Dutch braiding by taking the section of hair on the right and putting it *under* the middle section. Then take the section on the left and cross it underneath the section in the middle. As you continue braiding towards the back of your head, make sure to add new sections of hair to both your left and right strands.

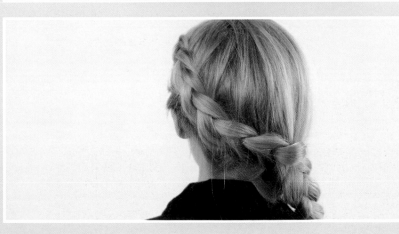

3. After all hair has been incorporated into the Dutch braid and you have braided all the way down to the ends of your hair, secure the braid with an elastic.

4. Tug lightly on each part of the braid to make it appear wider and more flared out.

5. Take your braid and form a spiral at the back of your head.

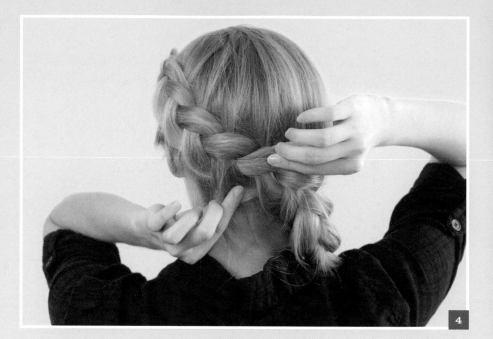

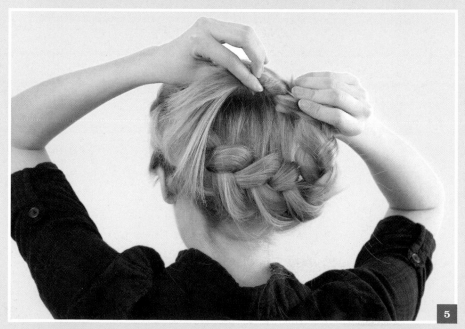

6. Tuck the unbraided ends of your braid into the spiral.

7. Secure the spiral with bobby pins.

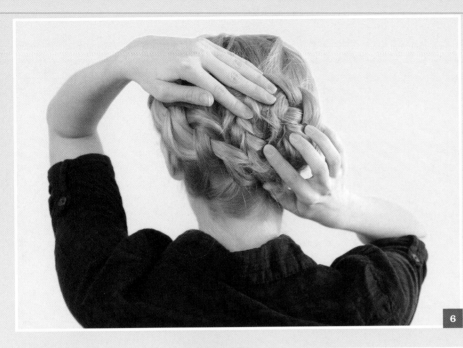

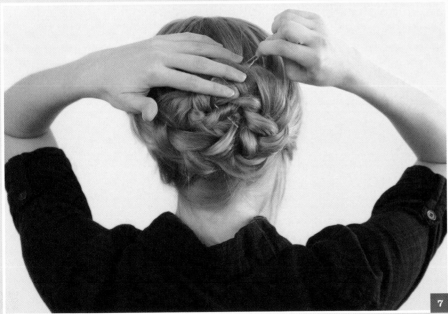

Milkmaid

Braid

Milkmaid braids make for a classic look that will never go out of style. Consisting of two Regular Three-Stranded Braids, this hairstyle is perfect for those just starting out with braids. Its adorable look can be pulled off by just about anyone and evokes a sense of folkish innocence wherever you go.

EASY

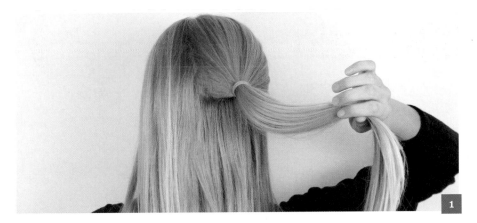

1. Section off the upper right quarter of your hair and pull it into a ponytail. Secure the hair with an elastic to get it out of the way.

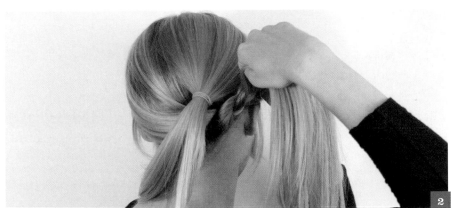

2. Sweep the hair from the left side of your head over to the right and begin braiding it upwards using the Regular Three-Stranded Braid technique. Make sure you include all loose, unbraided hair.

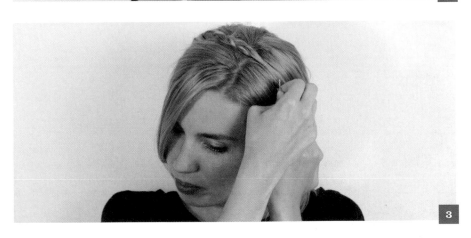

3. Braid until you reach the ends of your hair, then secure the braid with an elastic. Bobby pin the braid to the top of your head wherever you think it looks best.

4. Remove the elastic from the ponytail you created earlier and sweep the hair to the left side of your head. Begin braiding it upwards using the Regular Three-Stranded Braid technique. Once you reach the ends, secure the braid with an elastic.

5. Bobby pin the braid to the top of your head, making sure to tuck the ends of both braids under each other so that they aren't showing.

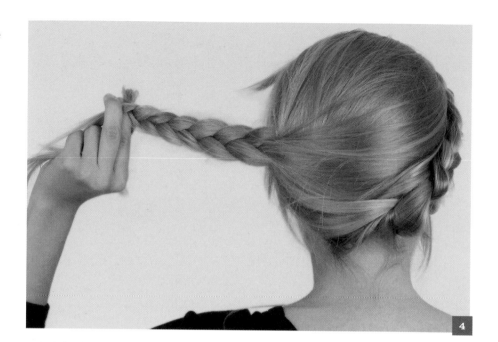

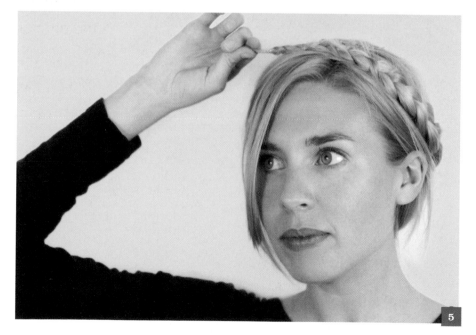

French Braid *Ponytail*

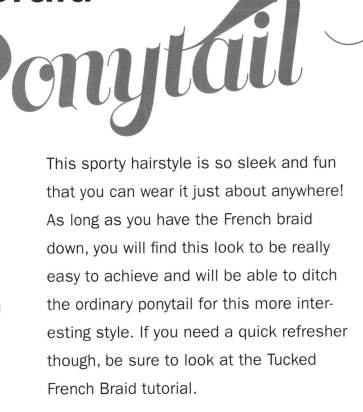

This sporty hairstyle is so sleek and fun that you can wear it just about anywhere! As long as you have the French braid down, you will find this look to be really easy to achieve and will be able to ditch the ordinary ponytail for this more interesting style. If you need a quick refresher though, be sure to look at the Tucked French Braid tutorial.

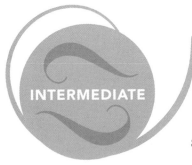

INTERMEDIATE

89

1. Take a small section of hair from the front of your head.

2. Begin French braiding this section by dividing the section into three smaller sections and crossing the right section over the middle section followed by the left section over the middle one.

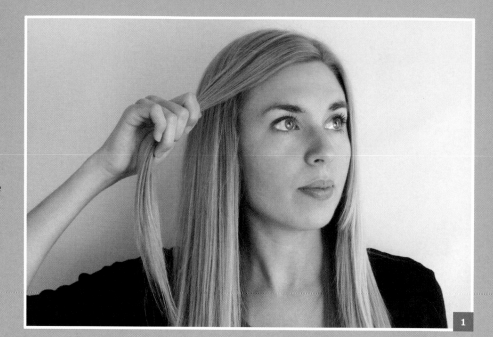

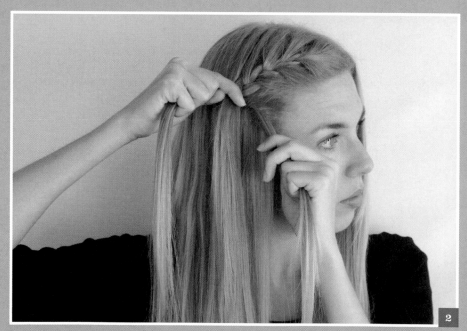

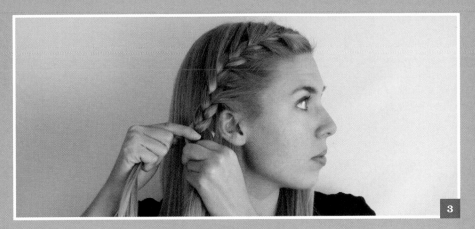

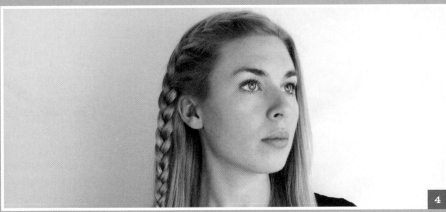

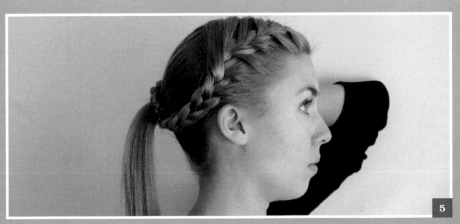

3. As you braid, make sure to gather new sections of hair and add them to the outer strands. Continue French braiding until you reach your ear and all of the hair closest to the scalp is incorporated into the braid.

4. Braid the remaining strands using the Regular Three-Stranded Braid technique and secure the braid with an elastic.

5. Pull your remaining hair into a ponytail. Wrap the end of your braid around the ponytail and secure with a bobby pin.

Braided *Crown*

Radiating elegance and beauty, the Braided Crown may make you feel like royalty. This regal design—made of two Lace Braids delicately pieced together—is a great look for special occasions, like weddings and baby showers, and will even make you feel sophisticated when you're not wearing a gown. If you haven't mastered a Lace Braid yet, it may be helpful to check out the tutorial found earlier in this book.

HARD

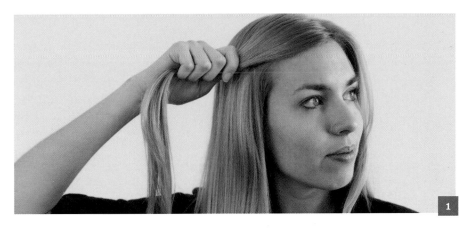

1. Gather a medium-size section of hair at the front of your head.

2. Divide the section into three pieces.

3. Begin creating a Regular Three-Stranded Braid by crossing the right section over the middle section.

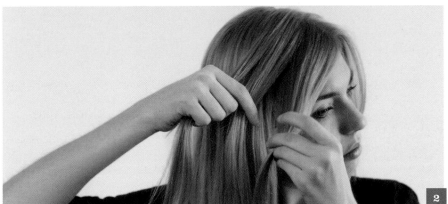

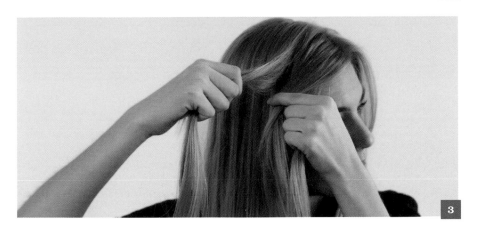

4. Cross the left section over the middle one.

5. Cross the right section over the middle section again without adding any additional hair.

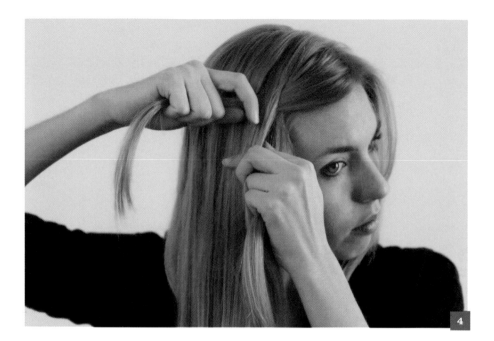

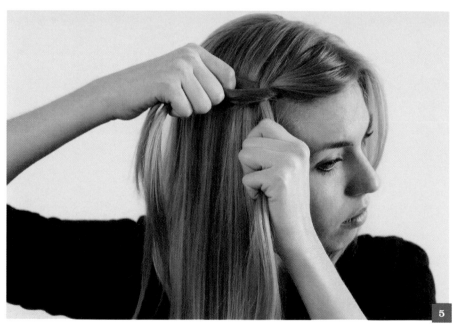

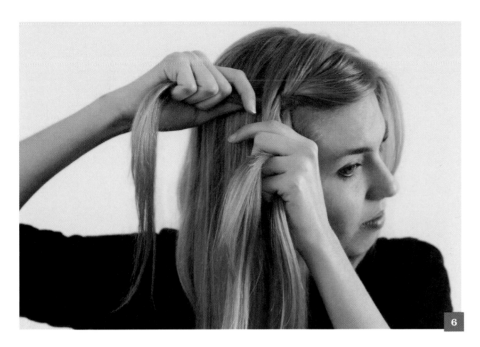

6. Add a small section of hair to your leftmost strand and cross this new section over the middle section.

7. Continue creating a Lace Braid until you reach the back of your head.

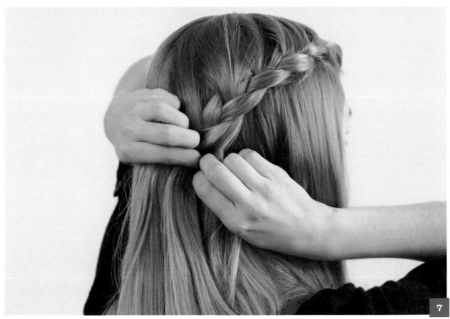

8. Secure the braid with an elastic.

9. Repeat Steps 1–7 on the other side of your head.

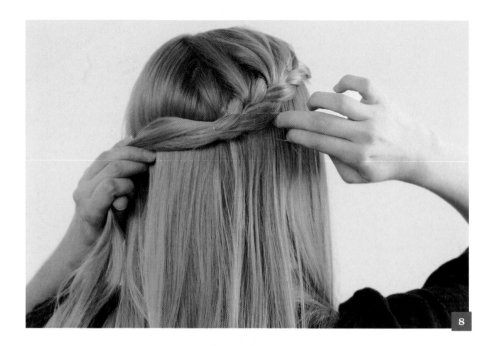

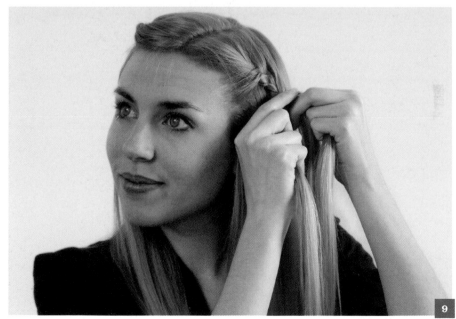

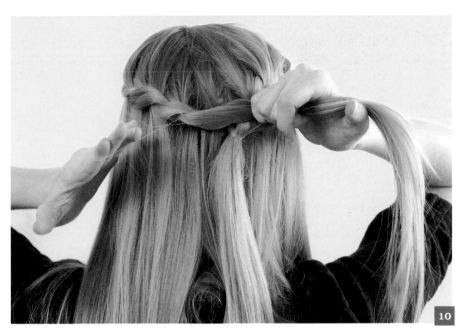

10. Secure the braid with an elastic.

11. Place the braids at the back of your head so that their ends touch. Secure them in place with a bobby pin.

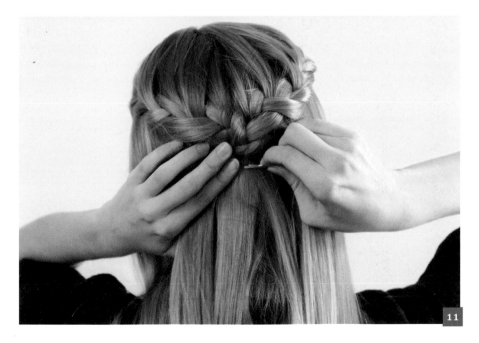

Double Lace *Braid*

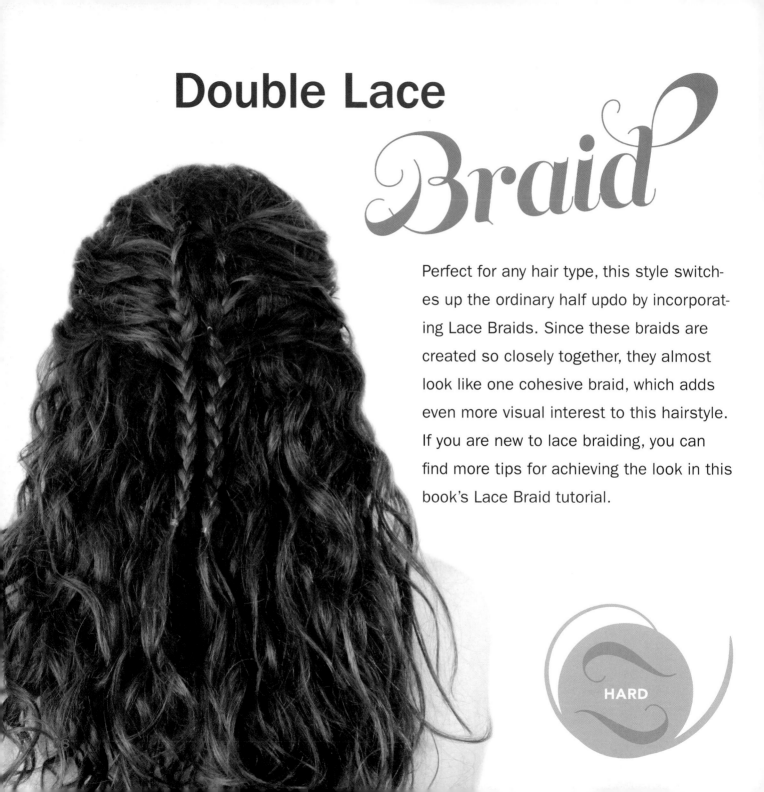

Perfect for any hair type, this style switches up the ordinary half updo by incorporating Lace Braids. Since these braids are created so closely together, they almost look like one cohesive braid, which adds even more visual interest to this hairstyle. If you are new to lace braiding, you can find more tips for achieving the look in this book's Lace Braid tutorial.

HARD

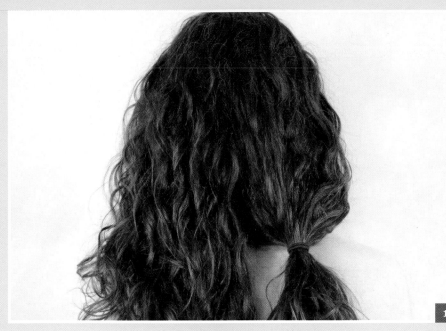

1. Start by parting your hair down the middle and creating two sections of hair at the back of your head. Secure the right section with an elastic to get it out of the way.

2. Braiding as close as possible to your part, start creating a Lace Braid using the remaining hair. You'll want to divide the left section into three smaller sections and cross the right section over the middle section. Then cross the left section over the middle one. As you continue braiding, make sure to add small sections of hair to your leftmost strand before you cross it over the middle section. Do not add any hair to the rightmost strand as you braid. When you have reached your ears, start braiding a Regular Three-Stranded Braid by

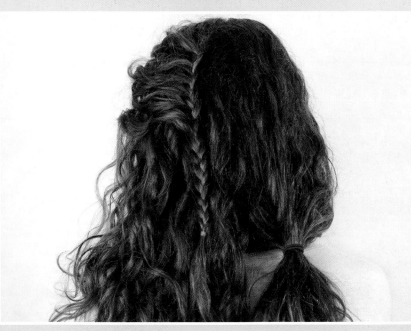

simply crossing the right strand over the middle and the left strand over the middle until you reach the ends of your hair. Secure the completed braid with an elastic.

3. Release your hair on the right side and repeat Step 2. When lace braiding on this side, however, make sure to add new sections of hair to the rightmost strand instead of the leftmost strand. Pull the braids closer together and secure them in place with bobby pins.

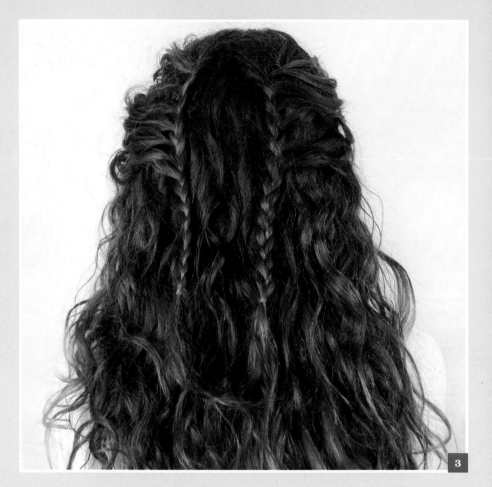

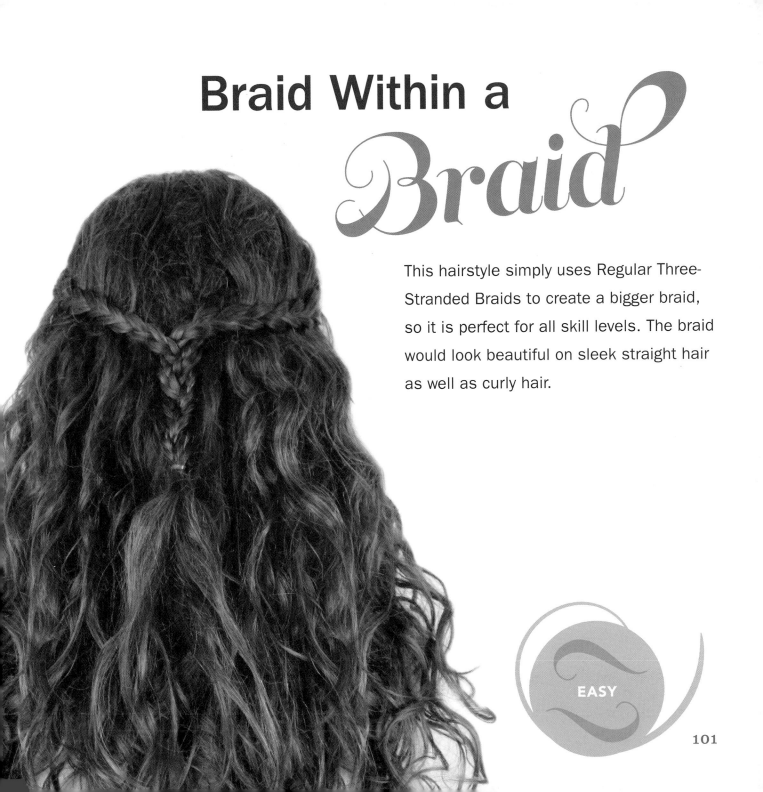

Braid Within a *Braid*

This hairstyle simply uses Regular Three-Stranded Braids to create a bigger braid, so it is perfect for all skill levels. The braid would look beautiful on sleek straight hair as well as curly hair.

EASY

1. Part your hair down the middle. Take a section from one side of your head and divide it into three smaller sections. Begin creating a Regular Three-Stranded Braid by crossing the rightmost section over the middle one and the leftmost section over the middle section. Continue braiding until you reach the ends of your hair and then secure the braid with an elastic.

2. Repeat the previous step on the left side of your head.

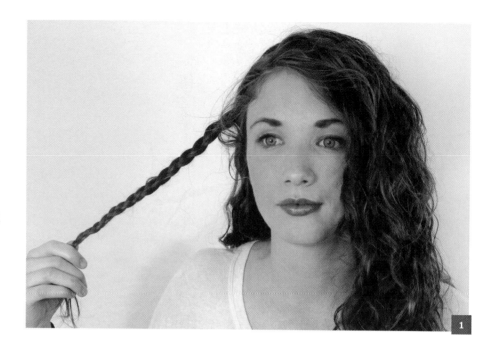

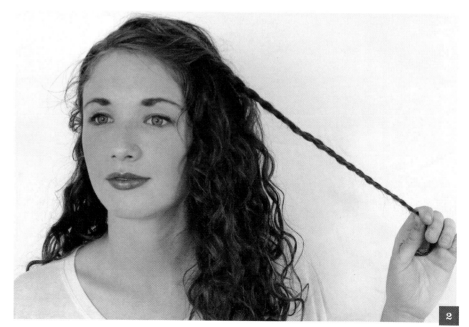

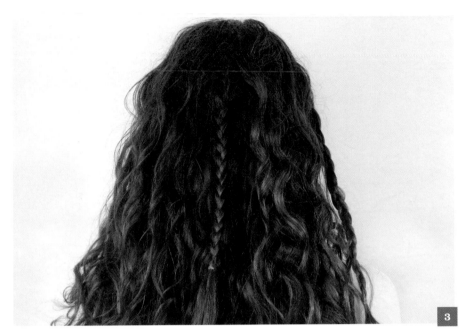

3. Gather a section of hair from the back of your head, just a few inches below the top of your head, and divide it into three sections. Repeat Step 1 using these sections of hair to create another Regular Three-Stranded Braid.

4. Braid the three braids together into a giant Regular Three-Stranded Braid by simply crossing the right braid over the middle one and the left braid over the middle section. Continue braiding until you have reached the ends of your hair. Secure the braid with an elastic.

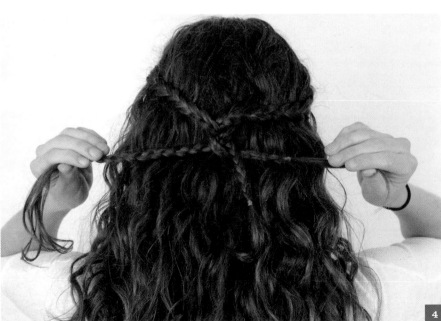

Side French 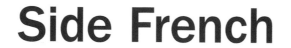 Braid

This French braid is unique compared to ones you typically see. It starts at your part and runs completely straight down just one side of your head. It's sure to get you lots of compliments, and is a fantastic look for the summer. This hairstyle utilizes French braiding so look back at the Tucked French Braid, if you are unfamiliar with this technique.

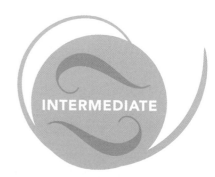

INTERMEDIATE

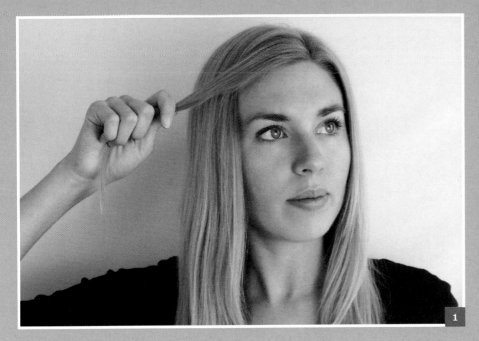

1. Gather a small section of hair at the front of your head.

2. Divide this section into three smaller sections and begin French braiding down towards the direction of your right ear. You'll want to cross the left section over the middle strands and then the right section over the middle strands, adding additional strands to the outer sections each time you cross them over the middle.

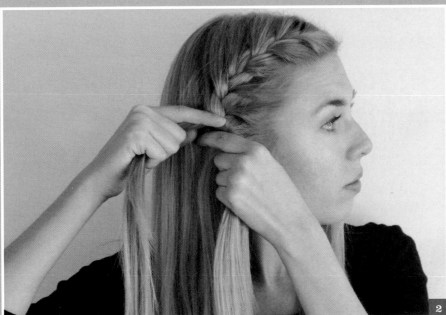

3. Once you reach your ear, begin grabbing small sections of hair from the other side of your head and incorporating them into the left side of the braid as you braid.

4. Continue braiding until you have reached the ends of your hair. Secure the braid with an elastic.

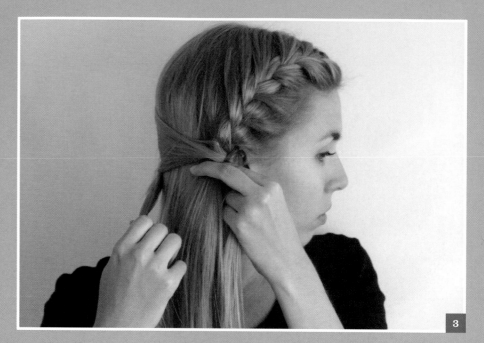

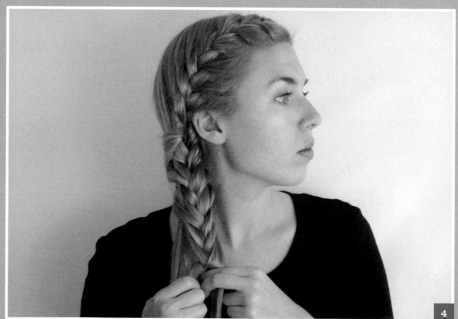

Faux Fishtail 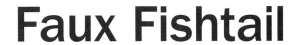 Braid

The Faux Fishtail Braid is great for those mornings when you hit the snooze button one too many times. It looks strikingly like a Fishtail Braid, but takes a fraction of the time and is less intimidating to those new to braiding. Another great thing about this do is that it is very sturdy so you will not worry about it falling out during the day.

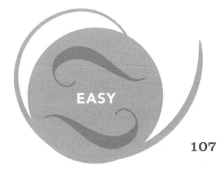

EASY

1. Pull your hair into a side ponytail and secure it with an elastic.

2. At the top of the elastic, divide the hair in half, forming a small hole.

3. Push the hair from your ponytail into the hole.

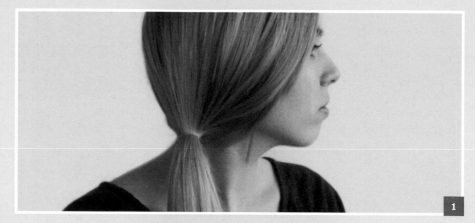

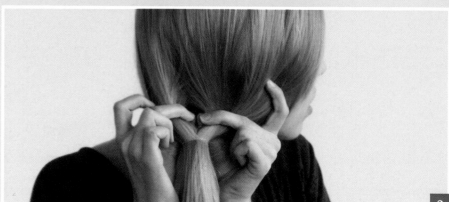

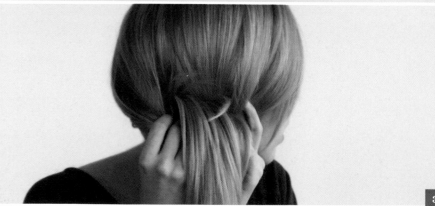

4. Bring the hair from your ponytail all the way through the hole.

5. Add another elastic a few inches below the first elastic.

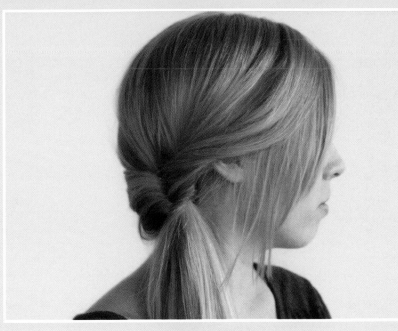

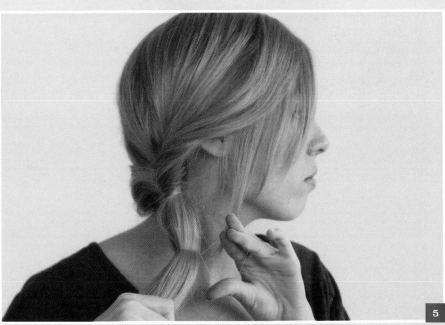

6. Repeat Steps 2–4 using the new elastic as a reference point.

7. If your hair is very long, you may want to repeat Steps 5–6 until you create a look that fits your hair's length.

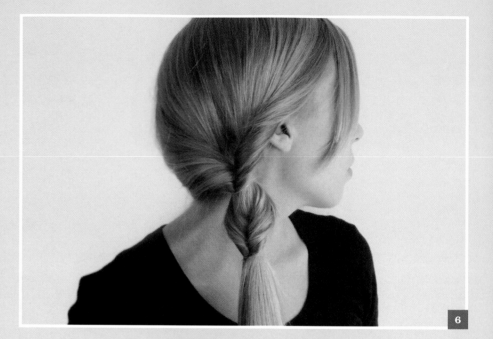

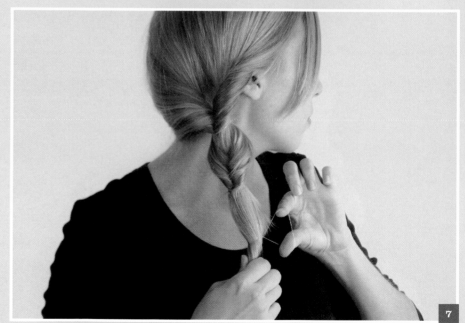

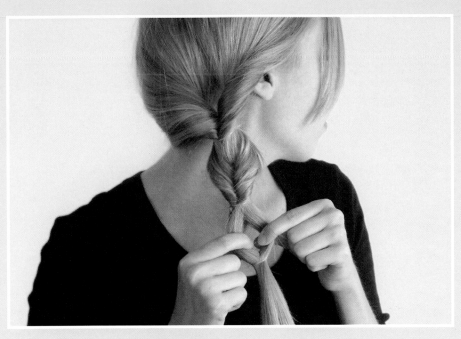

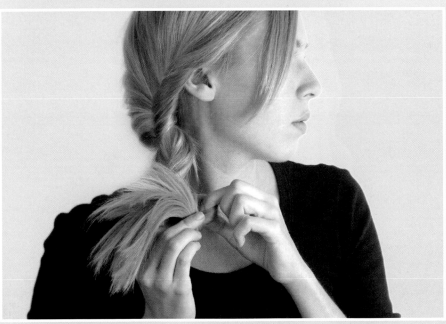

Figure 8 *Braid*

The Figure 8 Braid is another simple hair-style that can be completed in minutes. Al-though it's an easy braid to learn, it looks complicated, so you can look like a pro without having to put in too much work.

EASY

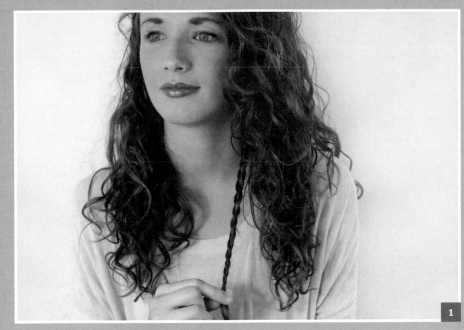

1. Take a small section of hair from the nape of your neck and divide it into three smaller sections. Begin a Regular Three-Stranded Braid by crossing the right section over the middle and then the leftmost section over the middle section. Continue braiding until you reach the ends of your hair and secure the braid with an elastic.

2. Divide the rest of your hair into two sections.

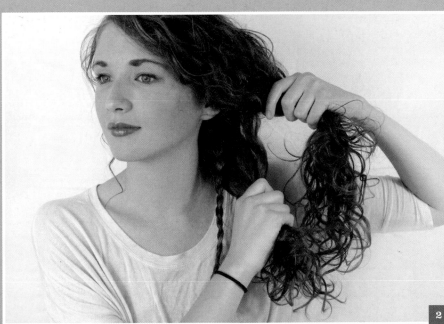

Figure 8 Braid 113

3. Cross the braid under the first section and over the second section.

4. Wrap the braid under the second section and over the first section. It should resemble a figure 8.

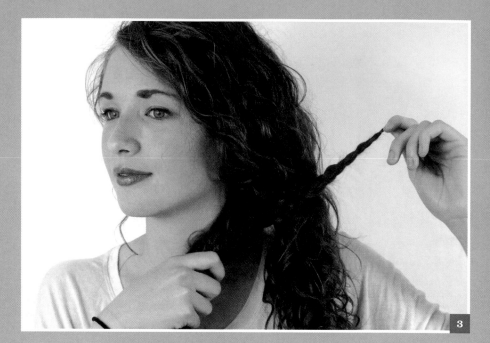

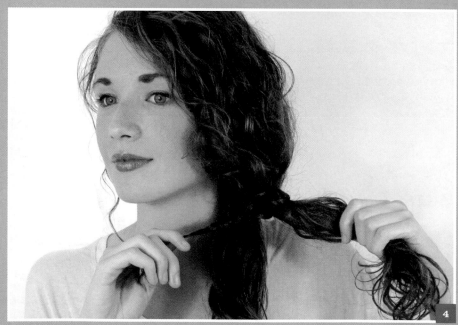

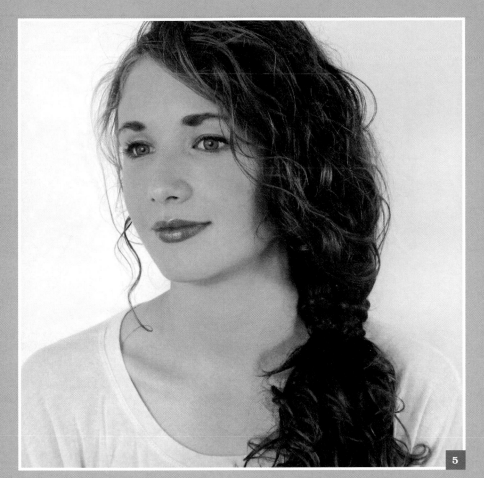

5

5. Using the same braid, repeat Steps 3–4 until you reach the end of your braid. Secure the braid with an elastic.

Figure 8 Braid   115

Dutch Braid

Bun

The Dutch Braid Bun is a difficult one to learn, but has quickly become a favorite among girls. Since the look includes Dutch braiding the underside of your hair until you reach the crown of your head, it can be tough to do to your own hair when you're just getting started. After some practice, though, you'll get the hang of it and will love showcasing the look at parties. For an in-depth description of Dutch braiding, look back to the tutorial for the Dutch Braided Headband.

HARD

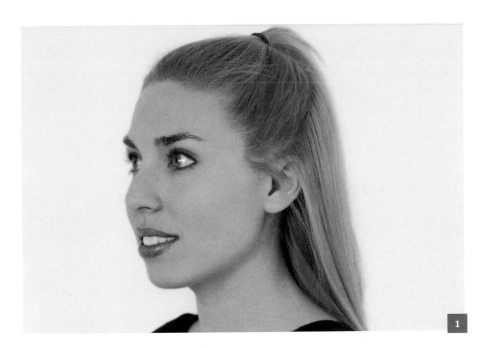

1. Pull the top half of your hair up into a ponytail on top of your head.

2. Turn your head upside down and gather a small section of hair closest to your neck. Divide this section into three smaller sections.

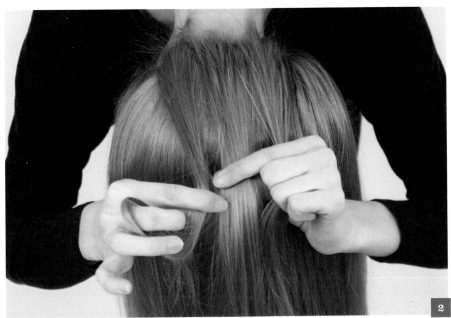

3. Start a Dutch braid by taking the section of hair on the right and putting it under the middle section. Then take the section on the left and cross it underneath the section in the middle. As you continue braiding, make sure to add new sections of hair to both your left and right strands.

4. Once you have incorporated all the free hair into the braid, secure the braid with an elastic.

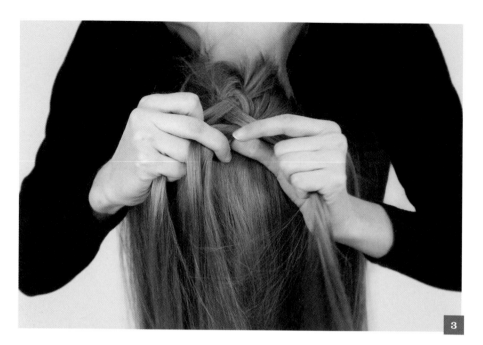

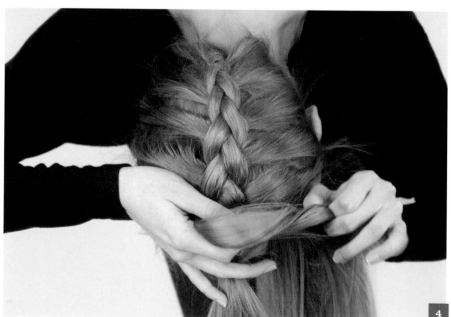

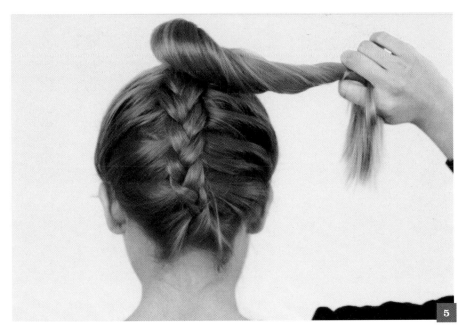

5. Return your head to its normal position and remove the elastic from the top portion of your hair. Gather this section of hair and add it to the braid. Your hair should make one large ponytail.

6. Twist the free hair and form it into a bun at the top of your head. Secure the bun in place with bobby pins.

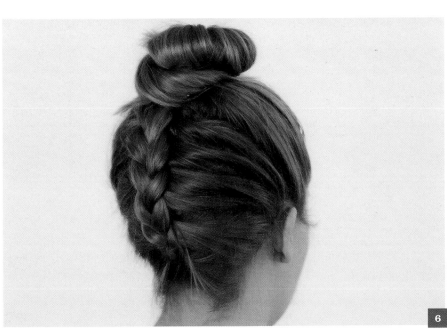

Four-Stranded
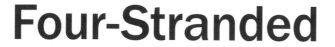

You may think you don't have enough hands for a Four-Stranded Braid, but it is not as hard as it sounds. The basic technique is taking the outside strand and weaving it under and over the other strands until you've incorporated all of your hair. The end result is a beautiful, complex-looking braid that will make people do a double take.

INTERMEDIATE

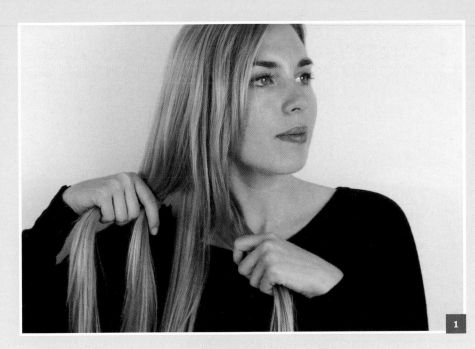

1. Divide your hair into four sections.

2. Cross the outer right section of hair, or moving section, over the section of hair closest to it.

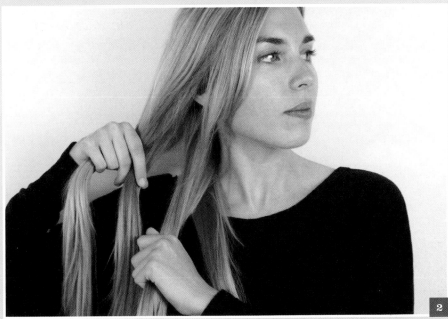

3. Weave the moving section under the next section of hair.

4. Cross the moving section over the last section of hair.

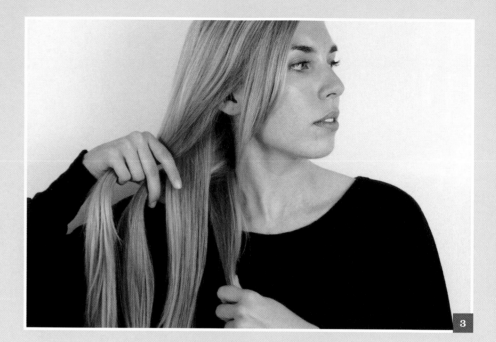

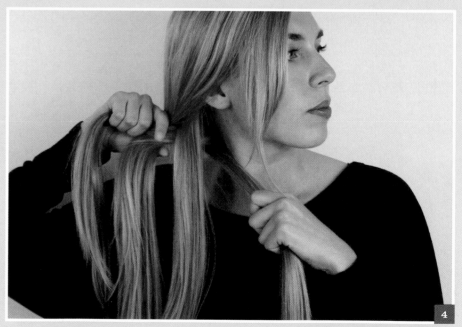

5. The section of hair that is now on the far right will become the new moving section and will be woven over and under the other sections in a similar fashion.

6. Repeat Steps 2–4 until you reach the ends of your hair. Secure the braid with an elastic.

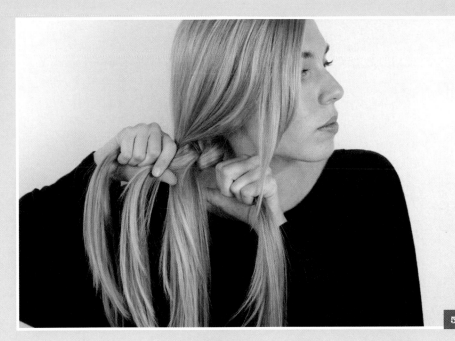

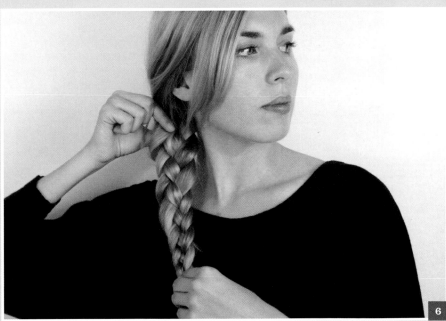

French Fishtail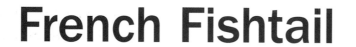

Absolutely stunning, the French Fishtail Braid is one of the more difficult braids to do on yourself simply because it takes a bit of time and can easily turn into a workout. Before starting this braid, be sure to understand the basics involved with creating a Fishtail Braid (instructions can be found earlier in the book). Again, with Fishtail Braids, always remember that the smaller the sections you use, the more beautiful and intricate the braid.

HARD

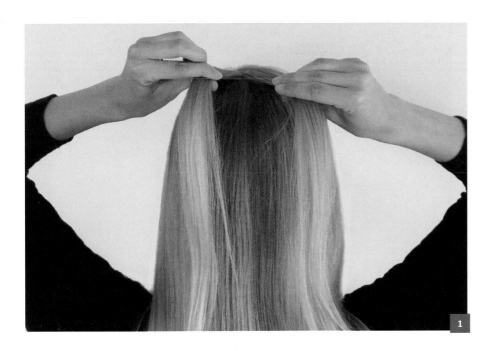

1. Take a section of hair from the crown of your head and divide it in half.

2. Take a small section of hair from the right side of your head, cross it over the rightmost crown section, and add it to the section of hair on the left side of your head.

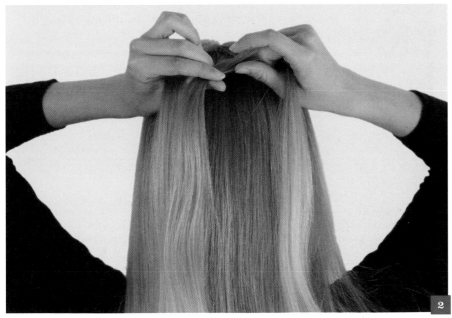

3. Take a section from the left side of your head, cross it over the leftmost crown section, and add it to the section on the right side of your head.

4. Continue to alternate adding new hair to the left and right sections until you reach the nape of your neck.

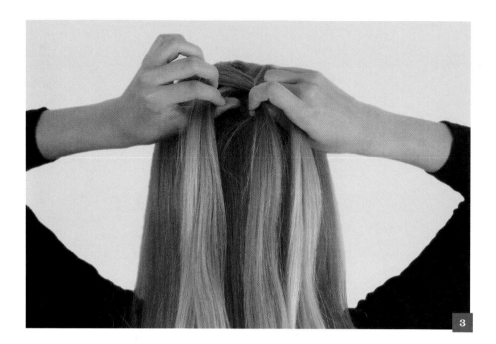

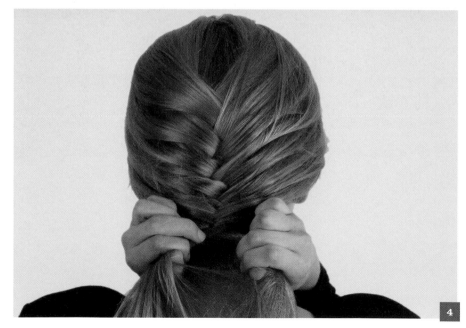

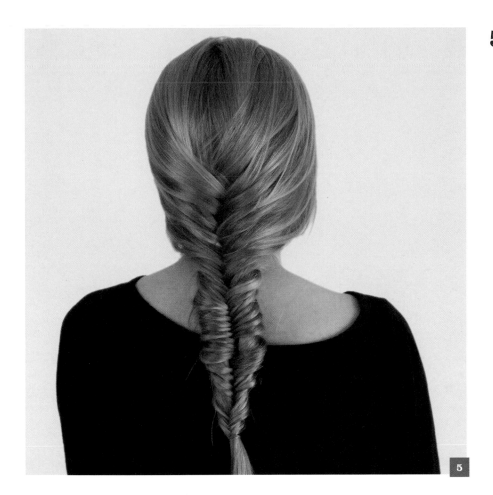

5

5. Once you have incorporated all your hair into the left and right sections, begin creating a regular Fishtail Braid. Take a small piece of hair from the right section and bring it over to the left section. Now take a small section from the left and bring it over to the right section of hair. Continue alternating sides until you reach the ends of your hair. Then secure your braid with an elastic.

Intertwined French *Braids*

This hairstyle looks like a complex arrangement of several braids intertwined together but, in reality, it is just two French braids that are strategically placed on your head. If you need a refresher on how to French braid, please see the Tucked French Braid tutorial. People often get intimidated about trying a style like this because it looks so complicated, but once you see the step-by-step breakdown you'll realize it's not as difficult as it seemed, and you'll be happy you gave this beautiful look a shot!

INTERMEDIATE

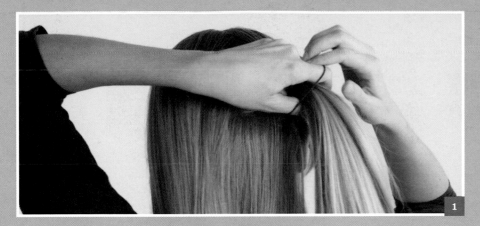

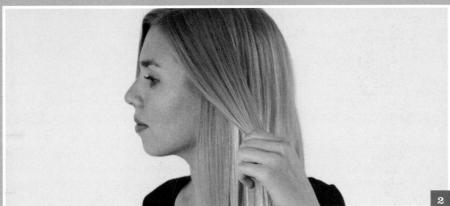

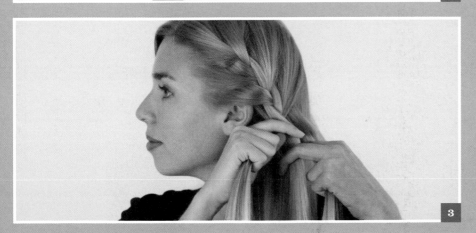

1. Gather a section of hair at the upper right quarter of your head and secure it with an elastic to get it out of the way.

2. Take a section of hair from the left side of your head, closest to the hairline.

3. Start creating a French braid by dividing the section into three smaller sections. Take the right section and cross it over the middle section, then take the left section and cross it over the middle section. As you continue braiding in this fashion, make sure to gather new sections of hair to add to the outer sections each time you cross them over the middle section.

4. Continue French braiding toward the bottom right corner until all of the hair closest to the scalp is incorporated into the braid.

5. Braid the remaining hair using the Regular Three-Stranded Braid technique and secure the braid with an elastic.

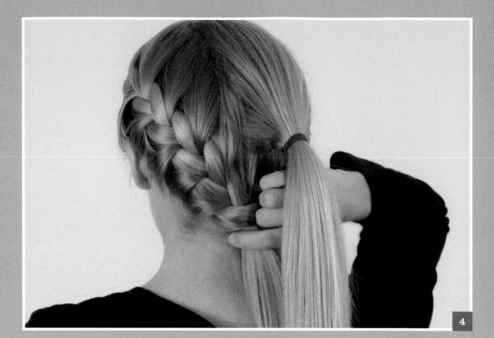

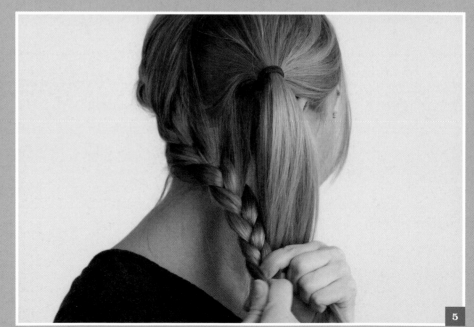

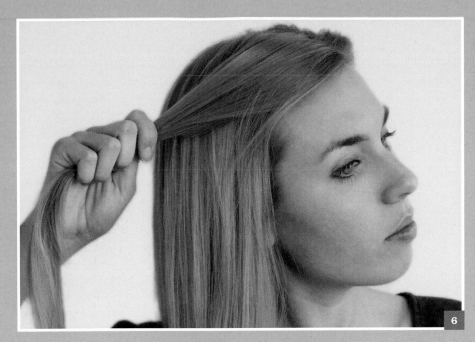

6. Remove the elastic from the section of hair at the top right of your head.

7. Repeat Steps 2–3, making sure to braid towards the bottom left side.

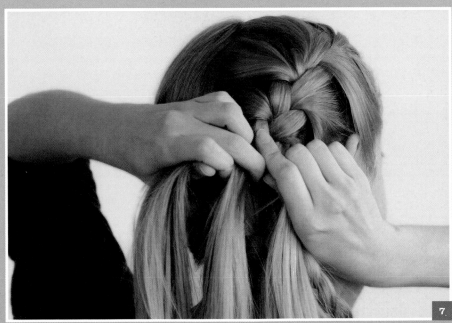

8. Once you finish braiding, secure the braid with an elastic. You should now have two French braids that crisscross in the back.

9. Use a bobby pin to secure the braid you just created behind your left ear.

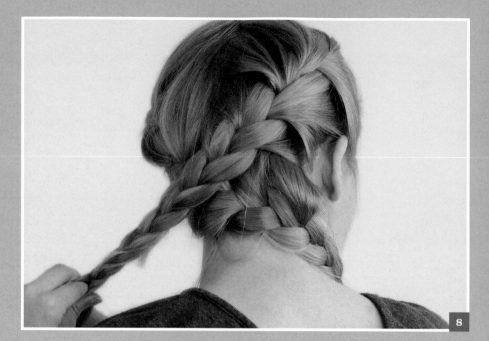

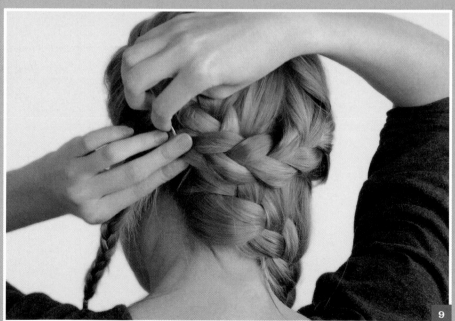

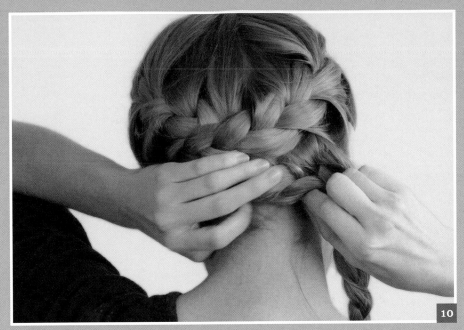

10. Bobby pin the rest of that braid underneath your right ear so that the ends don't show.

11. Take the braid hanging on the right side and arrange it so that it is now heading towards your left ear. Secure the braid with bobby pins and then pin the leftover pieces underneath the braid.

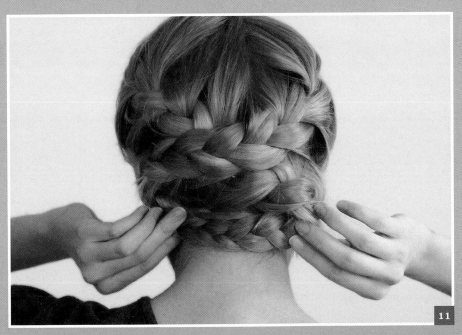

Intertwined French Braids **133**

Side French Rope *Braid*

The Side French Rope Braid is a fast and easy braid that wraps around the back of your head, making it beautiful from all angles. While it may be the perfect everyday look, this hairstyle is far from ordinary and will immediately grab the attention of onlookers. If you need a refresher on French Rope Braids, turn to the tutorial found earlier in this book for more detailed instructions.

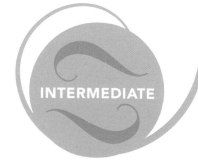

INTERMEDIATE

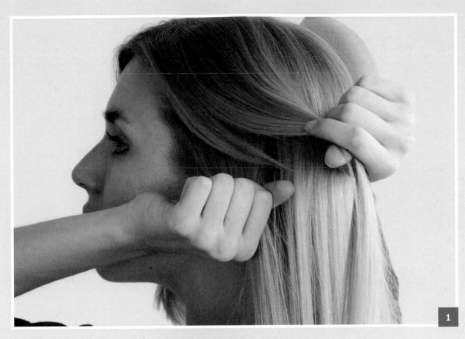

1. Start with two pieces of hair right above your ear.

2. Take the lower section and cross it over the section on top.

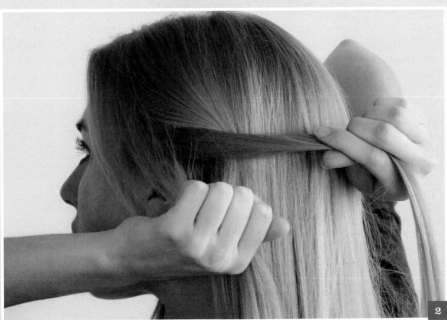

3. Add additional hair to the new lower section and cross it over the section on top.

4. Repeat the previous step until you have wrapped the braid around the back of your head and incorporated all your hair into the hairstyle.

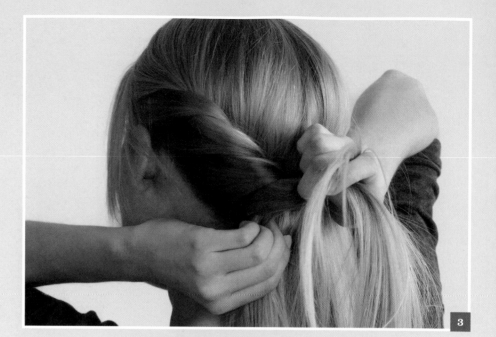

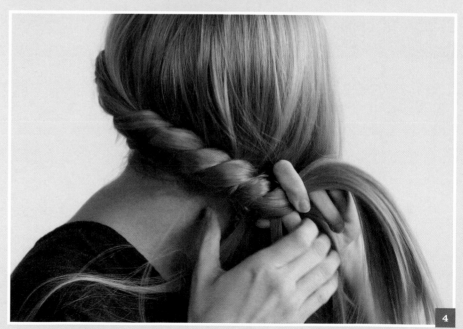

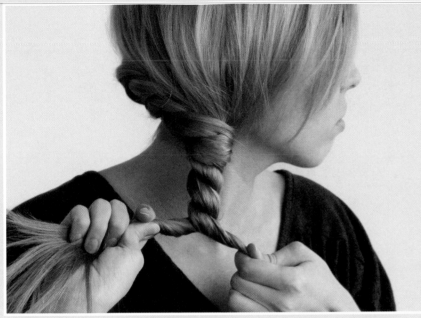

5. Once all your hair is in the rope braid and just right below your ear, twist both strands in the same direction and then wrap them around each other. Make the twists as tight as possible.

6. Secure the braid with an elastic. Keep in mind that the twist will loosen slightly but should remain intact.

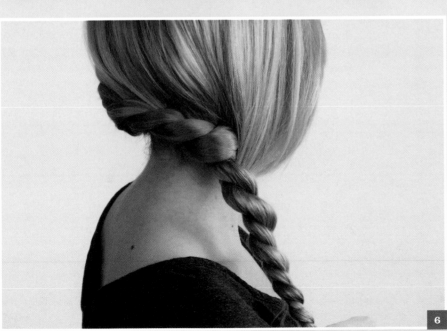

Skeleton *Braid*

Named for its rib cage–like appearance, the Skeleton Braid uses almost the same technique as the French braid, but adds a dramatic flair to the style. Because of its intricate design, this hairstyle will take a bit of practice and patience to achieve, but it's hauntingly beautiful when you're finished. It may be helpful when you're first starting out with the design to use a mirror to see the back of your head. Because this style uses a similar technique to the French braid, be sure to look back at the Tucked French Braid instructions before creating a Skeleton Braid.

INTERMEDIATE

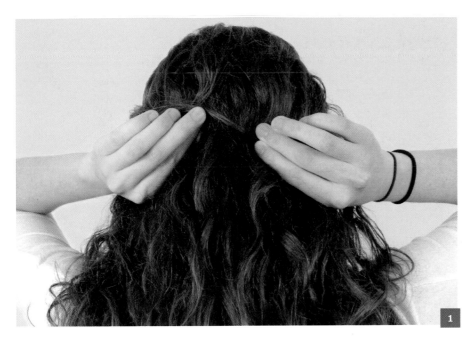

1. Gather three small sections of hair: one from the front left, one from the front right, and one from the crown of your head. Cross the left section over the middle one.

2. Cross the right section over the middle section.

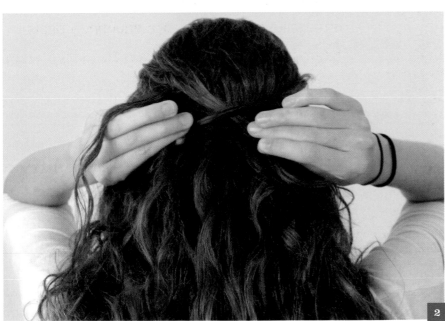

3. Gather a section of hair from the front left side of your head and add it to the leftmost section. Cross this new section over the middle section.

4. Gather a section of hair from the front right side of your head and add it to the rightmost section. Cross this new section over the middle section.

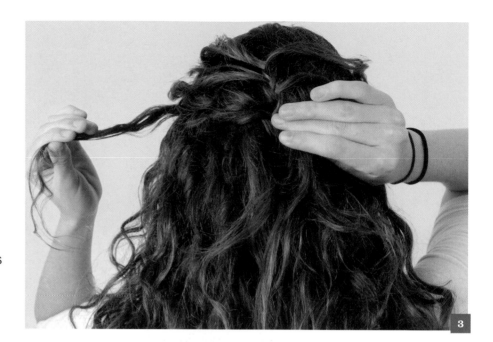

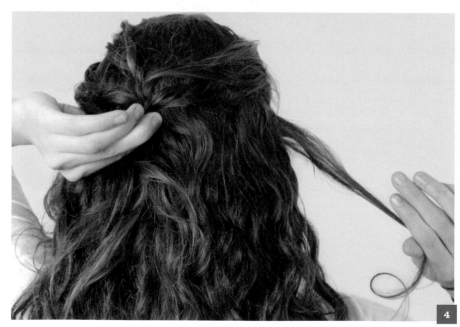

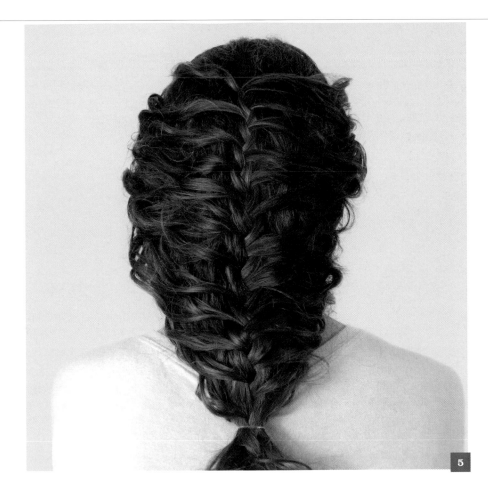

5. Repeat Steps 3–4 as far down as you would like the braid to go. Secure the braid with an elastic.

Triple Twist Braided

Buns

A versatile and sophisticated hairstyle, the Triple Twist Braided Buns could easily be taken from a casual, everyday look to a more formal event. It's another great beginner's hairstyle, so the only braid you'll need to know how to do beforehand is the Regular Three-Stranded Braid.

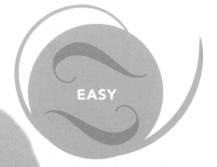

EASY

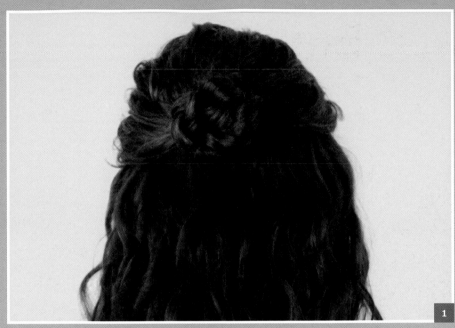

1. Gather the upper third of your hair into a ponytail. Loosely braid it to the ends using the Regular Three-Stranded Braid technique and secure it with an elastic. Slightly twist the braid once or twice into a bun at the top of your head and secure it with bobby pins.

2. Repeat the previous step one more time to create your second bun.

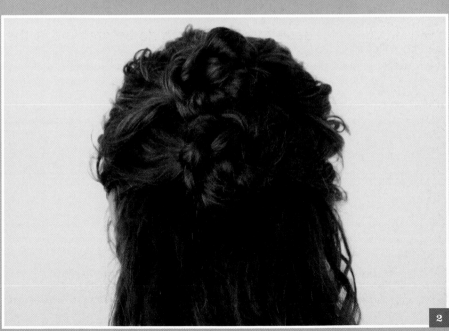

3. If you are happy with the look so far, you can leave your hair as is. You can also repeat Step 1 to create a third bun and complete the look.

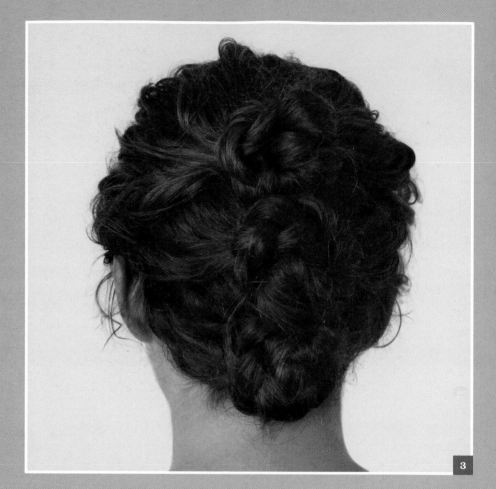

3